Pharmacy Calculations

An Introduction *for* Pharmacy Technicians

Joy Bellis Sakai, Pharm.D.

Clinical Pharmacist
Kaweah Delta Medical Center
Pharmacy Technician Training Program
College of the Sequoias
and
Partner
Rx Consultants
Visalia, California

Leanora Kasun, M.S.

Instructor
Redwood High School
and
Adjunct Instructor of Math
College of the Sequoias
Visalia, California

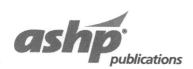

Any correspondence regarding this publication should be sent to the publisher, American Society of Health-System Pharmacists, 4500 East-West Highway, Suite 900, Bethesda, MD 20814, attention: Special Publishing.

The information presented herein reflects the opinions of the contributors and advisors. It should not be interpreted as an official policy of ASHP or as an endorsement of any product.

Because of ongoing research and improvements in technology, the information and its applications contained in this text are constantly evolving and are subject to the professional judgment and interpretation of the practitioner due to the uniqueness of a clinical situation. The editors, contributors, and ASHP have made reasonable efforts to ensure the accuracy and appropriateness of the information presented in this document. However, any user of this information is advised that the editors, contributors, advisors, and ASHP are not responsible for the continued currency of the information, for any errors or omissions, and/or for any consequences arising from the use of the information in the document in any and all practice settings. Any reader of this document is cautioned that ASHP makes no representation, guarantee, or warranty, express or implied, as to the accuracy and appropriateness of the information contained in this document and specifically disclaims any liability to any party for the accuracy and/or completeness of the material or for any damages arising out of the use or non-use of any of the information contained in this document.

Director, Special Publishing: Jack Bruggeman
Acquisitions Editor: Jack Bruggeman
Editorial Project Manager: Ruth Bloom
Editorial Resources Manager: Bill Fogle
Production Project Planner/Layout: Carol A. Barrer
Design: DeVall Advertising

We gratefully acknowledge the assistance of Dana H. Anderson, R.Ph., Director of Pharmacy and Sandy Brin, Inventory Control Technician at Virginia Hospital Center for their help in obtaining photos. We also want to thank Bryan Ashewood for his photography.

Library of Congress Cataloging-in-Publication Data

Sakai, Joy Bellis.
 Pharmacy calculations : an introduction for pharmacy technicians / Joy Bellis Sakai and Leanora Kasun.
    p. ; cm.
Includes bibliographical references and index.
ISBN 978-1-58528-261-6 (alk. paper)
I. Kasun, Leanora. II. American Society of Health-System Pharmacists. III. Title.
[DNLM: 1. Drug Dosage Calculations. 2. Pharmacists' Aides. QV 748]

615.1'9--dc23
                            2012016488

ASHP is a service mark of the American Society of Health-System Pharmacists, Inc.; registered in the U.S. Patent and Trademark Office.

ISBN: 978-1-58528-261-6

10 9 8 7 6 5 4

Dedication

This textbook is dedicated to math teachers everywhere (especially those who taught our kids). Although this subject is old, we know that to make it interesting requires original thinking, long hours, and sometimes even receiving telephone calls in the wee hours of the morning. So, thank you!

Joy Bellis Sakai and Leanora Kasun

Contents

Preface

As students enter into the study of pharmacy, they soon discover that it is a dynamic field where the roles of the pharmacist and pharmacy technician are continually evolving. This dynamism creates interest and opportunity for students who apply themselves. But even as the field changes, some things remain constant. The safety of patients is of paramount importance to anyone working in pharmacy, whether in hospital, retail, or institutional practices. A thorough understanding of basic pharmacy math and the ability to accurately perform computations continues to be a foundational skill for becoming the qualified, competent pharmacy technician that is always in demand.

This textbook is designed for pharmacy technician students enrolled in a training program, for technicians reviewing for the certification exam, and for on-site training in the workplace. It provides a complete review of the basic mathematics concepts and skills upon which a more advanced understanding of pharmacy-related topics must be built. Once the basic skills are reviewed, the student is guided through the pharmacy basics necessary for correctly interpreting prescriptions and drug orders and performing dosing calculations that technicians face in practice.

The goal in writing this text was to demystify pharmacy math, even for "math-phobic" students, by providing a stepwise approach from simple to complex pharmacy math problems built on a strong foundation of basics. After many years of teaching mathematics and pharmacy mathematics, the authors are aware that different students may connect with different approaches to math solutions. Therefore, when appropriate, different techniques for solutions are discussed.

Organization and Contents

The units and chapters of this text are organized to complement most pharmacy technician training curricula and to support the ASHP model curriculum. The chapters are divided into four units. Units progress from general and basic concepts to more specific and complex concepts.

- Unit 1, Review of Mathematics, provides an introduction to the world of pharmacy, including medication error avoidance. A complete review of foundational concepts and basic math operations follows, with an emphasis on how these concepts relate to pharmacy error prevention and patient safety.

- Unit 2, Systems of Measurement, reviews the metric system and introduces the apothecary system. Units encountered in pharmacy practice are discussed. Students are presented with conversions within and between measuring systems, and the application of dimensional analysis is taught. Temperature conversions and military time are covered here.

- Unit 3, Preparing for Problem Solving in Pharmacy, teaches students the basics of pharmacy abbreviations and prescription reading. The student will learn to calculate quantity to dispense and to verify a DEA number using the "checksum" digit. Basic algebra is reviewed. The unit covers estimation and a system for converting a word problem to an algebraic equation. Ratios are defined, and the use of the ratio and proportion system of problem solving is covered.

- Unit 4, Dosing Calculations and Other Pharmacy Problems, covers dosing calculations, percents, and concentration calculations, compounding formulas, and IV infusion calculations. The importance of using verified patient information for calculations and estimating before calculating is re-emphasized. Business terminology is defined and applications are explained.

Text Features and Additional Resources

Each chapter begins with clear learning objectives to help clarify the study approach at the outset. As students are introduced to pharmacy terminology, words and phrases are defined in the text. Term definitions in the margins create a natural way to find and learn new terms during study.

> **Drug Interactions**—The alteration of activity, metabolism, or excretion of one drug by another.

Key points are emphasized in the "Tech Note" highlighted boxes. This feature is designed to focus the reader's attention on important teaching points.

> **TECH NOTE!**
>
> *(1) A zero is always included to the left of the decimal point when writing a decimal fraction. (2) A zero is never included to the right of a decimal point.*

Each chapter provides multiple example problems with complete explanations. Examples move students from familiar, real-life problems to pharmacy-related problems.

EXAMPLE

Convert 2340 mg to g

SOLUTION ·

The new units (grams) are larger than the original units (milligrams), so divide to convert. One gram is 1000 mg, so divide by 1000, or move the decimal point three places to the left.

2340 mg = 2.340 g

Practice problems are found at the end of every chapter. Accurate solutions to odd-numbered problems are at the end of the text. Text appendices include the parts of a prescription, glossary of terms, and conversions and abbreviations tables.

Instructors will appreciate the additional resources found online through the ASHP web site. Resources include notes on the chapters for the instructor, more practice problems, and answers to all the problems. Instructors will also find ideas for extending chapter content through critical thinking questions and in-classroom activities (available at www.ashp.org/techcalculations). Suggestions for connecting math content to other areas of the pharmacy technician curriculum are provided for each chapter.

The authors and the ASHP publication team have worked hard to create a user-friendly math textbook that is accurate and covers the breadth of possible pharmacy math problems that a pharmacy technician might face. We are interested in hearing from our users and invite your feedback. Write to: The American Society of Health-System Pharmacists, 7272 Wisconsin Avenue, Bethesda, MD 20814, attention: Special Publishing.

Acknowledgments

We wonder what springs to most people's minds when they think of writers. Perhaps someone with paper and pencil, sitting in an easy chair near a sunny window, gazing out on a pastoral scene, while the perfect sentence springs from the writer's imagination to the page? We hate to burst any bubbles, but writing is more like a team relay race, where the book gets passed back and forth, is written, rewritten, and illustrated, all while running toward a finish line. Writing isn't for sissies, but thanks to teamwork, it can be an interesting and fulfilling process.

We want to thank our entire team at ASHP, including the two people who originally got us started on the project, Rebecca Olson and Dana Battaglia. Many thanks go to our editorial reviewers, who provided great suggestions for improvement. Most especially, thanks to Ruth Bloom and Bill Fogle who, in spite of joining the team late, got us over the finish line in record time.

Last, but certainly not least, thanks to our husbands and families who supported us with patience and dinner on numerous occasions. Having said how much help we got from the team, we need to state that any errors in the text are our responsibility.

Joy Bellis Sakai and Leanora Kasun

Reviewers

Lynn Breegle, B.A., C.Ph.T.
Program Instructor
Chaffey College
Rancho Cucamonga, California

Mark Brunton, C.Ph.T.
Program Director
Kaplan College
Las Vegas, Nevada

Marlene Lamnin, R.Ph.
San Leandro Hospital
Castro Valley Adult and Career Education
Castro Valley, California

Elina Pierce, C.Ph.T., MSP
Program Chair
Southeast Community College
Lincoln, Nebraska

Review of Mathematics

CHAPTER 1

Welcome to the World of Pharmacy

LEARNING OBJECTIVES

1. List three different settings where pharmacy is practiced.
2. Describe two duties of retail and hospital pharmacy technicians and the math skills they require.
3. List four factors that may contribute to medication errors.
4. List four important work habits technicians should employ to reduce the risk of making medication errors.

**UNIT
1**

Introduction

Although many people express discomfort with mathematics and avoid it as though it was a disease, math avoidance is something that no one starting on a career as a pharmacy technician can stick with for long. Math is nothing to be afraid of, and in fact, when a comfortable relationship with mathematics is developed, it can assist in many day-to-day activities. You use math every time you get change back from a cashier, calculate gas mileage, or figure out if you have enough money to buy all the groceries you need.

In the first chapter of this book, you will learn a little about the world of pharmacy, and the important role of math in that world. As a pharmacy technician, you will play an important role, too. Pharmacy is the profession that is responsible for managing a patient's medication use, and pharmacists are the professionals to whom pharmacy technicians report. Pharmacists assure that patients receive the most appropriate medication to meet their needs, and must consider many patient specific factors in order to make that determination. A patient's height, weight, age, and drug allergies are just some of the factors that are reviewed by the pharmacist before a prescription or drug order is filled. In order to successfully deliver the right product, the prescription or drug order must be filled accurately, in the correct dose, and for use at suitable intervals, while avoiding **drug interactions**, side effects, and other pitfalls associated with medication use.

Drug Interactions—The alteration of activity, metabolism, or excretion of one drug by another.

Pharmacy Practice Settings

Most pharmacies, whether in a hospital, retail, or other setting, are very busy places; in fact they can at times be downright chaotic. The technician is asked to take on much of the repetitive work in a pharmacy so that the pharmacist can spend his or her time with cognitive functions; that is, assuring that each patient gets the appropriate drug.

Outpatient—A patient whose illness is cared for at home.

Compound—Preparation of a product from pharmaceutical-grade ingredients to meet the needs of the patient.

Reconstitute—To bring a medication to the liquid state by the addition of water or another diluent.

Retail pharmacies

Retail pharmacies provide prescription services to **outpatients**, people who are taking care of illness from their own homes. Retail pharmacy technicians collect important data from patients (age, height, weight, allergies), prepare labels, weigh, measure, and **compound** medications, all while answering telephones and fielding and referring questions from customers or health care professionals.

In order to function effectively in this kind of setting, technicians must be able to read a prescription, including Roman numerals and Latin prescription abbreviations. Sometimes technicians are called upon to convert measurements from the apothecary or household systems of measurement to the metric system. Technicians in retail practice settings **reconstitute** oral medications and assist customers with selecting measuring devices to measure oral liquid medications, so understanding measurements of solids and liquids is important.

Because a retail pharmacy is a business, technicians will need to understand concepts associated with discounts and mark-ups, and costs and profit margins. A thorough understanding of percentage calculations will make your life as a retail pharmacy technician easier. Business mathematics uses the same mathematical operations, but has its own vocabulary, with which a retail pharmacy technician needs to be familiar.

NUMBERS AT WORK
Retail pharmacy is a business that requires technicians to understand business concepts and business mathematics. An understanding of discounts, mark-ups, margins, and percentage calculations are important for a technician's success in the retail environment.

Hospital pharmacy practice

Although many of the duties of the hospital and retail pharmacy technician overlap, there are some significant differences. Essentially every hospital pharmacy compounds sterile products for intravenous injection. As you will see, products given intravenously carry a greater risk to the patient and require a wider range of skills on the part of pharmacy staff members. Hospital pharmacy technicians need to learn sterile compounding vocabulary, techniques, and use of special equipment. This type of work also requires a facility with reconstitution, dosing calculations and flow rate problems. You will find chapters on dosing, reconstitution, and flow rates near the back of the book. Once you work your way through earlier chapters, you will be prepared for these more advanced problems.

Other pharmacy practice settings

Some pharmacy technicians work in specialty pharmacy practices, such as compounding pharmacies, long-term care pharmacies, or home **infusion** pharmacies. Compounding and home infusion pharmacies specialize in non-sterile and sterile compounding, respectively. In these settings, most of the technician's day will be consumed with weighing, measuring, and preparing compounded products. Knowing how to reduce and enlarge formulas is essential for this work, as are dosing calculations.

Infusion—The slow, continuous introduction of a solution, especially into a vein.

In long term care pharmacies, medications are often distributed to nursing homes in quantities to last 1 month. Technicians must be able to read prescriptions and calculate the number of tablets, capsules or liquid medication to assure that the patient has the supply of medicine he or she needs. Knowledge of business math is important in this setting because technicians may be processing bills for insurance companies or other **third party payers**.

When you have a thorough understanding of the ins-and-outs of pharmacy math problems, you will be able to adapt that knowledge and understanding to new problems as they arise. It is not enough to be able to plug numbers into formulas. You must be able to see the logic of a problem in order to avoid mistakes. As important members of the pharmacy team, it is crucial for technicians to solve math problems with confidence. By routinely using safe medication practices like double-checking, getting clarification when in doubt, estimating, and always staying focused on the patient, you can help avoid medication errors.

Third Party Payers—A company, organization, insurer, or government agency that makes payment for health care services received by a patient.

The Problem of Medication Errors

Authorities at the Institute of Medicine believe that medication errors may be responsible for harming as many as 1.5 million people each year and may cost 3.5 billion dollars annually due to death, injury, or extended hospitalization.[1] These errors occur for any number of reasons, including improper storage, prescribing, dispensing and administration of a drug. However, a significant number of errors occur because of miscalculation of doses or miscalculation made during the compounding of a drug.

Unfortunately, it is children that are very often the victims of dosing calculation errors. This is partly because children cannot receive drugs on a one-size-fits-all basis. Medication doses for children are calculated based on their weight or body surface area. Children from the ages of newborn to 18 years of age are considered pediatric patients, and can range in weight from 1 kg (or 2.2 pounds, not unusual for a premature infant) to 100 kg (220 pounds, not unheard of for a 16-year-old male). Clearly, pharmacists and technicians must be very careful when calculating pediatric doses because if the decimal point gets put in the wrong place there is the potential for a ten-fold dosing error.

 NUMBERS AT WORK
Dosing calculations for babies and children are especially problem prone. Always double check the patient's weight and have a pharmacist check pediatric calculations.

Consider the case of one small, but healthy, 3-year-old boy. His physician ordered IV arginine, a drug used to test production of growth hormone, but instead of supplying the 5.75 grams of arginine ordered, the outpatient pharmacy sent 60 grams, a 10-fold error. Even though his mother expressed concern to the nurse and physician about the effects the drug was having, the child received the entire 60-gram dose. He was admitted to the hospital that night and died shortly thereafter. The error that caused this child's death was preventable, as are all dosing errors.

Becoming a Good Pharmacy Technician

In any human undertaking, there is a potential for errors to occur. Although mistakes will never be completely eliminated, we know that there are factors that contribute to errors in health care, as in any other area. People who are distracted, tired, or are working in a stressful environment are more likely to make errors. Health-care workers who do not follow accepted safety policies, or assume that someone else's work is correct without actually checking it, are likely to make errors. When a serious error is made, the person responsible carries a tremendous burden forever, and in effect becomes the "second victim" of the error. As you start out in pharmacy, establish works habits that will make you a better and safer technician.

> **TECH NOTE!**
>
> *Establish work habits now that will make you a better technician later.*

In order to avoid causing a medication error, a technician must have a clearly legible drug order or prescription. The technician should have a basic understanding of the medication and its uses. Is the drug very toxic or relatively safe? It is essential that you know certain facts about a patient before beginning a dosing calculation. Is this calculation for a child or an adult? How much does the patient weigh? What is a typical dose for an adult? If the drug is for a child, are the calculations based on the correct weight?

Of course, whenever you, as a technician, make a calculation, you must have the pharmacist check it. It helps to get in the habit of double-checking your own answers, and having another technician check them, too. Most importantly, every time you calculate a dose, estimate it first and listen to your instincts. Does your answer make sense, or does it require you to prepare an unusually large volume, or use multiple vials, tablets or capsules for the patient? When pharmacy staff, nurses, and physicians take the time to ask and answer these questions about medication use, errors can be avoided.

Accuracy and precision

In day-to-day conversation the terms accurate and precise are sometimes used interchangeably. There is a difference, however, and an understanding of both words is important in the field of pharmacy. **Accuracy** means the closeness of a measurement to its true value, while **precision** refers to the reproducibility of a measurement over many different operations. When applied to work, a person that performs consistently accurate work would be described as precise. Hopefully, every pharmacy technician student will strive to be precise.

As you work through this text, remember how important you will be in the lives of the patients you serve. If you have had "math phobias" in the past, it is time to put them behind you. Pharmacy math is not difficult, but it is crucial, and to master it you must put in the necessary time and practice. Try to work all of the math problems without looking at the answers, and learn how to look for the information you need to answer problems. As the student, we ask that you work to develop a feel for the processes, learn the metric system, memorize abbreviations and conversions, and do the problems. With these tools, and learning to always

Accuracy—The closeness of a measurement to its true value.

Precision—The ability of a measurement to be consistently reproduced.

estimate first and then double-check your work, you will become a welcome addition to the practice of pharmacy.

To maximize your success while learning pharmacy math, familiarize yourself with the appendices and other important information within this text. The following questions are designed to help guide you to areas of the text you will need during your course of study.

The most important job of anyone who works in pharmacy is to assure that every customer or patient receives the appropriate medication, whether it is a prescription medication or a drug purchased over-the-counter. Working the practice problems at the end of this and every chapter will help prepare you to safely undertake that work. Remember, the best way to become proficient at anything is practice, practice, and more practice!

UNIT
1

Practice Problems

1. Use the appendix to answer the following questions about prescriptions and drug orders:
   a. What is a "sig"?
   b. What does "Rx" mean?
   c. Where is information about the prescriber usually found?

2. Find the list of Latin prescription abbreviations to define the following abbreviations:
   a. PO   b. PRN   c. IV   d. QHS

3. Where are the learning objectives for each chapter located?

4. Find the glossary and define the following terms:
   a. Adverse drug event   b. Drug interaction   c. Compound

5. Use the Internet to find the body surface area of a 5-year-old boy who is 45 inches tall and weighs 40 pounds.

6. Why is it important to know the age and weight of a person before performing a dosing calculation? Write a sentence or two to explain.

7. Why do you think it is important to know what a medication is used for before you fill a prescription for it? Write a sentence or two to explain.

8. An adult male weighs 75 kg. Use the Internet to find his weight in pounds. Does he weigh more in pounds or in kilograms?

9. Use the Internet to find a case report of a serious dosing or calculation error. Write up a paragraph on the error and include the following:
   a. What was the cause of the error?
   b. What was the age of the person injured?
   c. Were there procedures or practices that contributed to the error?
   d. How might it have been prevented?

Reference

1. Preventing Medication Errors: Quality Chasm Series, National Academies Press. Available at: http://www.nap.edu/catalog.php?record_id=11623. Accessed December 22, 2011.

CHAPTER 2

Numbers and Numerals

LEARNING OBJECTIVES

1. Define *number*.
2. Define *numeral*.
3. Apply the rules for the use of Roman numerals to convert an Arabic numeral to a Roman numeral, and a Roman numeral to an Arabic numeral.
4. List an example of an integer, whole number, fraction, and decimal fraction.
5. Name the place value of the three digits to the left and the right of the decimal point.

Introduction

We use math every time we get change back from a cashier, calculate our gas mileage, or figure out if we have enough money to buy all the groceries we need. People who work in pharmacy must be especially confident in their understanding of numbers, basic math operations, and problem solving using basic algebra. In pharmacy, we must calculate doses, convert from one measuring system to another, and weigh and measure accurately in order to prepare safe and effective medications for patients.

People uncomfortable with mathematics may finish high school feeling relieved that they will never have to take another math class. However, if we who work in pharmacy do not develop our pharmacy math skills and practice them, we put patients' lives at risk. Because an understanding of numbers, number systems, and basic mathematical functions are the underpinnings for every math operation we perform in pharmacy, the first chapters in this text are devoted to a review of these concepts.

Numbers and Numerals

What is a number?

Humans have been counting since prehistoric days, as evidenced by scratch marks left on pre-historic artifacts. Even some animals have "number sense," the intuitive understanding of the relationship between numbers and things. The concept of "number" is one of the most basic concepts in science and mathematics. Yet the notion of number is difficult to define, because it is abstract. A number has no meaning except when it is used to count or measure a member of a group of similar things. For example, you can say you went to the grocery store for 10 apples, or a pound of fruit, and be understood. But if you say you went to the grocery store for 10, and don't define the purchase, the person you are speaking

Number—A label for counting or measuring objects or members of a set.

to is going to be confused. For the purposes of this text we will use the following definition of number:

> ▶ **TECH NOTE!**
>
> *A number is a label for counting or measuring things that are members of a definable set.*

So, how does this apply to our use of numbers in pharmacy? What this means is that we must always be aware of what we are counting or measuring. In pharmacy, a number alone, without information about what units are attached, is worse than useless, it is dangerous.

EXAMPLE

Nurse Watters, a new nurse, received the following order for Betsy Ross:

| 7/15 | Give Lasix 20 IVP x 1 now |
| | James Chalmers, M.D. |

She wondered whether she should fill the order with 20 mg or 20mL. How should Nurse Watters proceed?

SOLUTION

When a confusing or incomplete order is received, a nurse or pharmacist must call to clarify it. In this case, Nurse Watters proceeded to draw 20 mL of Lasix into a syringe and gave it to Betsy. When Mrs. Ross became ill, Nurse Watters' error became apparent. The usual dose of Lasix is 20 mg, not 20 mL (200 mg).

If we understand and apply the rules of mathematics when we work with numbers, errors are prevented. In the case of Nurse Watters we see that if she had been aware of the importance of units, she would have checked with the physician instead of making an invalid assumption, and would have avoided the resulting overdose.

Mathematics is a system for conveying information about numbers, in a simple and effective way. When the rules of math are consistently followed, the results of problems will be accurate. Mathematics communicates information in a way that transcends language barriers. Of all the specialized tools and equipment used in pharmacy, a working mastery of basic mathematics may be the most important.

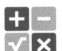

NUMBERS AT WORK

In the pharmacy as in every area of life, a number is meaningless without defining to what it relates. Units of measurement must always accompany a number to avoid dosing errors.

What is a numeral?

While a number is a label for counting or measuring members of a definable set, a numeral is the written symbol for that number.

> **▶ TECH NOTE!**
>
> *A numeral is a written symbol used to represent a number.*

Numeral—A written symbol used to represent a number.

There are many systems of numeration, but the system used by most of the world is the Arabic system, with numerals 0,1,2,…9. Most people are also aware of Roman numerals, a system we became familiar with in grade school and rarely used again. The Roman numeral system was widely used in prescription writing in the past. Physicians used this system, along with Latin abbreviations, in order to obscure the meaning of prescriptions. Although we live in a more enlightened age where the hope is that patients will understand their prescriptions, there is some carryover of the use of Roman numerals, so it is important for technicians to understand how these numerals work.

The numerals used in the Roman system appear in Table 2-1. We follow certain conventions, or rules, for the use of this system. As it turns out, even the Romans did not adhere strictly to the rules applied to the use of Roman numerals today, but without some sort of system, errors would follow. Table 2-2 is a summary of Roman numeral conventions.

Table 2-1. Numerals Used in the Roman System

Roman Numeral	Arabic Numeral
I	1
V	5
X	10
L	50
C	100
D	500
M	1000

Table 2-2. Rules for Interpreting Roman Numerals

1. Roman numerals are written in order from largest to smallest value, and each succeeding number is added to reach a total.

   Example: The Arabic number 11 is written: XI = 10 + 1 = 11

2. Numerals can be repeated up to 3 times. These are added together to reach a total.

   Example: XXX = 10 + 10 + 10 = 30

3. When a smaller numeral is written before a larger numeral, you subtract it from the larger numeral. You cannot repeat the same numeral and subtract it twice.

   Example: IX = 10 – 1 = 9

   IIX ≠ 8

4. Only I, X, and C are used for subtraction (not V, L, or D), and these numbers are only used in front of numerals that are 10 times their value or less.

   Example: IX = nine, but IC cannot be used for 99.

   99 is written XCIX.

5. Although the usual convention with Roman numerals is to use uppercase, in pharmacy lower case letters are often used. Lower case ss is considered = 1/2.

   Example: iss = 1½

Number Systems

Perhaps because humans have 10 fingers and 10 toes, it is very convenient to group numbers by tens. Although mathematicians and computer scientists are comfortable using other number systems, in everyday life we use the base 10, or decimal number system. When we count things, we use natural numbers. Natural numbers are whole numbers greater than zero that continue sequentially forever, or infinitely.

Rational and real numbers

Whole, or natural numbers, are not adequate for the work done in pharmacy. Just as you may only want a half sandwich for lunch, prescribers may need patients to receive a part of a tablet or vial of medication. Fractions and whole numbers are what are called rational numbers, or numbers that can be expressed as a ratio of two **integers**. An integer is any number that is not a fraction, whether positive or negative. A ratio is expressed as A/B, where A is any integer and B is any integer except zero. If B (the denominator) is equal to one, the ratio is an integer. If B is greater than one, the ratio is a fraction. If A (the numerator) is zero, then the ratio is equal to zero. If either A or B is less than one, the ratio is a negative number. Therefore, we can say that the rational numbers include all whole numbers, fractions, zero, and negative numbers.

An irrational number cannot be represented as a simple fraction (a ratio of integers). Pi (3.1415…) is an example of an irrational number. Pharmacy math problems are concerned with the rational numbers, whole numbers, fractions and zero. Figure 2-1 shows the relationship between different types of numbers.

Integer—Mathematical term to define the set of whole numbers both positive and negative, as well as 0.

Figure 2-1. Relationship among numbers.

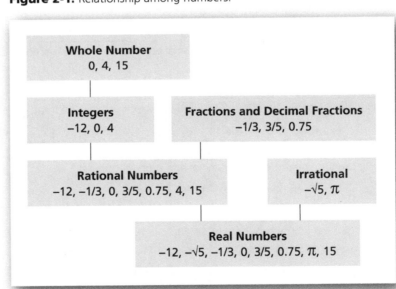

Place value

One important advantage of using a decimal system becomes apparent when we consider place value. **Place value** is a system of notation where the position of a numeral with respect to a reference point determines its value. In the decimal system, each place is a multiple of ten, and the reference point is called the decimal point.

Numerals to the left of the decimal are whole numbers beginning with the unit, or ones, position and increasing in value by multiples of 10. Numerals to the right of the decimal are fractions, with each place becoming smaller by divisions of 10. Decimal fractions are covered in more detail in Chapter 3.

In pharmacy, correct multiplication and division of decimals, and understanding of place value is crucial to avoid ten-fold under- or overdosing when we calculate doses. It is important to follow two rules for writing numerals with decimal points.

> ### ▶ TECH NOTE!
>
> *(1) A zero is always included to the left of the decimal point when writing a decimal fraction. (2) A zero is never included to the right of a decimal point.*

This is referred to as a **leading zero.** When the leading zero is not used in a handwritten drug order, the decimal point can be missed and the order misread (see Figure 2-2). Similarly, a **trailing zero** is never used in pharmacy, because it, too, can be misread and cause a ten-fold dosing error.

Place Value—A system of notation where the position of a numeral with respect to a decimal point determines its value.

UNIT 1

Leading Zero—A zero to the left of the decimal point, used in health care to prevent misinterpretation of drug strengths less than one.

Trailing Zero—A zero in the decimal representation of a number, after which no other digits follow.

Figure 2-2. Decimal place value. Notice that numbers to the right of the decimal are fractions, while those to the left are whole numbers.

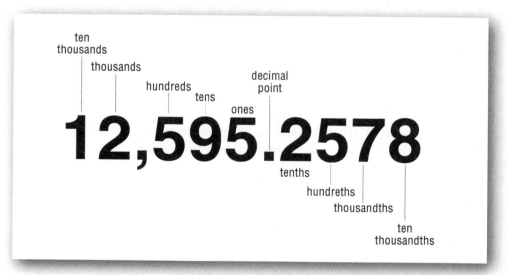

Example 1

It's easy to misread a handwritten medication order when the drug strength is written without a leading zero, such as:

digoxin .25 mg

The correct and safe way is to write:

digoxin 0.25 mg

Example 2

Here is how an order with a trailing zero might look. Imagine how unclear the decimal point might be if it were a faxed copy:

Lorazepam 2.0 mg

The correct, safe way to write this order is:

Lorazepam 2 mg

Rounding numbers

When solving a pharmacy math problem, answers may include decimal fractions with four or more digits to the right of the decimal point. Depending on the units in the problem, these fractions are likely to be unmeasurable with the equipment available in most pharmacies. In these instances, the technician or pharmacist must round the answer to a measurable volume or quantity. Unmeasurable digits are considered insignificant digits.

When using equipment such as a syringe or graduated cylinder, the precision of the measurement depends on the divisions marked on the device. For example, a 10-mL syringe is normally marked in divisions of two tenths of an mL (0.2 mL). In pharmacy practice, it is considered acceptable to measure an amount no smaller than one half the volume marked by division lines on the measuring device you are using. On a 10-mL syringe, then, volumes would have to be rounded to the nearest tenth of an mL (0.1 mL). See Figure 2-3.

Imagine that in calculating a drug dose, you find that you need to measure 425 mg of the antibiotic vancomycin. You notice that the concentration of the vancomycin in the vial is 100 mg/1 mL. You determine that the volume you need to measure is 4.25 mL. (You will learn to set up and solve this kind of problem in future chapters.) A 10-mL syringe is the appropriate sized syringe for measuring this volume of liquid. The question is, can you accurately measure a volume of 4.25 mL when the syringe is marked in 0.2-mL increments? Because the last digit, 0.05 or 5/100 is smaller than 0.1 mL it cannot be measured precisely. Therefore, the volume must be rounded.

When rounding, first determine the number of digits you will need in your answer. Perform the calculation, and locate the last digit you want to keep in your answer. If there is an additional digit to the right and it is 5 or more (a 5,6,7,8, or 9) you will increase the value of that last digit by one. If the number to the right of your last digit is 4 or less, you will leave the last digit as it is.

In situations where you need to round to the nearest five or ten, determine whether your answer is more or less than halfway to that number. If it is less than halfway, round down and more than halfway, round up.

Figure 2-3. A 10-mL syringe is marked with 0.2-mL increments.

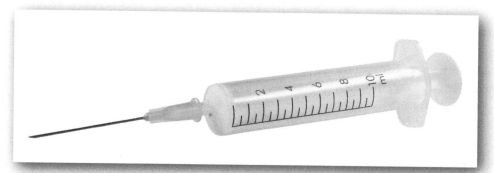

EXAMPLE

Joan calculates that she needs to measure 118.9 mL of distilled water to re-constitute the antibiotic suspension for baby Joseph Davis. The 150-mL glass graduate that is available for measuring is marked in 10-mL increments. How should Joan round the volume needed?

SOLUTION ··

Joan knows she can measure in 5-mL increments only (halfway between the 10-mL division lines); therefore, she will need to round to the nearest 5 mL. Her initial calculations were for 118.9 mL. She knows that her options are to either round down to 115 mL or up to 120 mL. Since 118.9 is more than half-way between 115 and 120, she will round up to 120 mL.

Practice Problems

In pharmacy, Roman numerals are most likely to be encountered when reading a prescription. Convert the following pharmacy-related examples as directed in the problem. Refer to Appendix A (Parts of a Prescription), and Appendix C (Latin Prescription Abbreviations and Medical Terminology), for more information.

1. Convert these Roman numeral volumes to Arabic numerals:
   a. iv fluid ounces   b. viii oz   c. XII oz

2. The following Roman numeral notations might be found in the sig, or directions, of a prescription. Write the amount so a patient could read it.
   a. iss tsp   b. ii tsp   c. iii drops

3. On a prescription, some prescribers write the number of tablets or capsules to be dispensed as Roman numerals. Write the following Arabic numerals as Roman numerals:
   a. 120 tablets   b. 36 capsules   c. 24 tabs

4. Convert the following Arabic numeral volumes or quantities to Roman numerals:
   a. 3 tsp   b. ½ fl oz   c. 5 mL

5. Write these Roman numeral prescription quantities as Arabic numerals. The abbreviation "disp" means dispense.
   a. Disp # XLV   b. Disp xxviii tablets   c. Disp xvi oz

Answer the following problems about place value:

6. Write the place value names for each digit in the following decimal fractions:
   a. 0.125 mg   b. 0.5 mL   c. 0.375 g   d. 0.02389 g

7. Write the place value names for each digit in the following whole numbers:
   a. 4   b. 55   c. 675   d. 12, 463

Round as directed in the problem.

8. Round the following to the nearest tenth:
   a. 11.674   b. 22.449   c. 100.39   d. 49.73

9. Round the following to the nearest 0.5 mL:
   a. 122.9 mL   b. 1.4 mL   c. 0.72 mL   d. 17.6 mL

Complete the following word problems:

10. Patrick is measuring salicylic acid for compounding an ointment. He calculates that he needs to measure 2675 mg of salicylic acid, but the balance (weighing device used in pharmacy) can only measure in increments of 10 mg. How many milligrams should Patrick weigh?

11. René Norris needs to measure 3.5 mL of Augmentin 600 for her toddler Joe's ear infection. She has a 5-mL oral syringe, marked in 0.2-mL increments. Can she accurately measure 3.5 mL in the 5-mL syringe?

12. Dr. Leland calculates that his patient needs a dose of phenobarbital, based on body weight, of 144.58 mg to be given twice a day. Phenobarbital is available in a concentration of 4 mg per mL, so you will need to draw up 36.145 mL for each dose. A 60-mL syringe has 1-mL calibration markings.

   a. To what volume should you round in order to measure as accurately as possible?

   b. Should Dr. Leland be contacted to make this change in the order?

13. Patsy Pitts, the pharmacy technician at Save Rite Pharmacy, receives a prescription as follows:

   Promethazine with Codeine
   Disp: viii fl oz

   She sees a 16-fluid ounce bottle that appears to be about half full on the shelf. How many ounces of promethazine with codeine will be left after the prescription is filled?

14. Rich Mann is trying to figure out how much medication to dispense for the following prescription:

   Prednisone 1 mg/mL
   Disp: 10 day supply
   Sig: 3 mg (3 mL) p.o. daily

   How much prednisone will Rich dispense in order to provide 10 days' worth of medication?

15. Jenny Jones, C.Ph.T., prepares discharge medications for patients going home from the hospital's surgery center. She receives a discharge prescription with the following Rx:

   Vicodin tablets
   Disp # XLVIII

   She has only one bottle of 100 tablets left and has another prescription for 24 tablets. If she dispenses the Vicodin as ordered here, will she have enough left to fill the second prescription?

In the following examples there are problems in the way these prescriptions or drug orders are written. List the errors and explain why they are dangerous.

16, 17, 18. There are three examples of error-causing practices in the way the prescription below is written. Based on what you learned in this chapter, identify the problems and explain why they could be dangerous to the patient.

Beatrice Heinz, M.D.
1200 Du LacPlace
Lakeside, Minn

Name: Anne DeLong   Date: 1/1/12
Address: 1248 Saint Cloud Drive, Lakeside

Rx: Levothyroxine 125.0
        Disp: XXXX

Sig: One tablet P.O. daily

Refills: 0 1 2 3   Beatrice Heinz   M.D.

19, 20. The pharmacy department received the following drug order. Find the two problem-prone writing practices in this order and explain why they are dangerous.

Morphine Sulfate 2 IV Q 2 hours prn pain. If patient becomes overly sedated give Narcan .4 mg SC q 15 minutes prn excess sedation, up to 3 doses.

Review of Basic Math Operations

LEARNING OBJECTIVES

1. Add, subtract, multiply, and divide whole numbers.
2. Simplify fractions.
3. Find a least common denominator.
4. Add, subtract, multiply, and divide fractions and mixed numbers.
5. Convert fractions to decimal fractions.
6. Add, subtract, multiply, and divide decimal fractions.

Introduction

There are four operations, or ways of performing a calculation, in mathematics: addition, subtraction, multiplication, and division. No matter how complicated a calculation is, it will only involve some combination of these four operations. In this chapter you will have a chance to refresh your memory on the vocabulary and rules that apply to these math basics.

Addition and Subtraction

Two numbers that are added are called **addends**. The answer to an addition problem is called the sum or the **total**. In a word problem, when you see that the answer calls for a sum or total, it is a clue that addition is required for the solution.

Addend—A number that is added to another number.

Total—The answer to an addition problem.

EXAMPLE

Carl and Mary were in the pharmacy compounding the IV piggyback bags for the afternoon delivery. Mary made 44 piggyback bags and Carl made 27. How many IV piggybacks did they make in total?

SOLUTION ···

Mary made: 44 bags
Carl made: + 27
Total: 71

When two numbers are subtracted, the result is called the **difference**. When a word problem asks for an answer with more, less, or the difference between two numbers, it is an indication that subtraction will be used.

Difference—The answer to a subtraction problem.

Factor—That which is multiplied.

Product—The answer to a multi-plication problem.

Prime Number—A number (other than one) whose only fac-tors are one and itself.

Quotient—The answer to a divi-sion problem.

Divisor—A number by which another number is to be divided.

> **EXAMPLE**
>
> How many more IV piggyback bags did Mary make than Carl?
>
> **SOLUTION** ·
>
> 44 bags – 27 bags = 17 more bags

Multiplication and Division

Numbers that are multiplied together are called **factors**. The result of a multi-plication problem is called a **product**. As you will see later in this chapter, when performing mathematical operations on fractions, it is important to be able to find the factors that make up a given number.

> **EXAMPLE**
>
> Identify the factors in 21
>
> **SOLUTION** ·
>
> The factors are 3 and 7, because
>
> $$3 \times 7 = 21$$

> **EXAMPLE**
>
> Find the product 8 × 7
>
> **SOLUTION** ·
>
> $8 \times 7 = 56$

A number whose only factors are one and itself is called a **prime number**. The number one is not considered a prime number. Here is a list of the first several prime numbers:

$$2, 3, 5, 7, 11, 13, 17, 19, 23, 29$$

When numbers are divided, the result is called the **quotient**. The number be-ing divided is called the dividend, and the number that is being used to divide is called the **divisor**. Division can be written several different ways.

> **EXAMPLE**
>
> How many ways can we write the problem 10 divided by 5?
>
> **SOLUTION** ·
>
> $$10 \div 5 = 2$$
>
> Dividend   Quotient
>
> Divisor
>
> or
>
> Divisor $\longrightarrow$ $5)\overline{10}$ $\longrightarrow$ Quotient
>
> Dividend

or

Dividend ⟶ $\dfrac{10}{5}$ = 2 ⟶ Quotient

Divisor

When using a calculator to calculate a quotient, the dividend is always entered first.

EXAMPLE

Find the quotient.

a. 15 ÷ 3

b. $\dfrac{20}{10}$

c. $9\overline{)63}$

SOLUTION

a. 15 ÷ 3 = 5

b. $\dfrac{20}{10}$ = 2

c. $9\overline{)63}^{\,7}$

Sometimes the divisor does not go evenly into the dividend and we have some quantity left over, that is, a remainder.

EXAMPLE

Pharmacy technician Hugh Morris must repackage 465 tablets into bottles containing 20 tablets each. How many bottles are needed and how many tablets will be left over?

SOLUTION

$20\overline{)465}^{\,23}$ Remainder 5

So, 23 bottles will be needed with 5 tablets left over.

Working with Fractions

A fraction consists of a numerator (the top) and a denominator (the bottom) separated by a fraction bar. The numerator indicates the portions and the denominator indicates how many portions make a whole. For example, in the fraction ¾, the numerator "3" tells how many portions, and the denominator "4" indicates that four 4ths make a whole, or one unit. Figure 3-1 uses a pie to represent how a whole can be divided into equal portions.

The fraction bar is interpreted as a division symbol, so a fraction is really a kind of division problem. A fraction may also be interpreted as a ratio, or a relationship between two numbers.

> **TECH NOTE!**
>
> *A ratio is the relationship between two quantities.*

Figure 3-1. If a pie is cut into eight equal pieces, the whole pie could be described as 8 eighths, or 8/8. If one person eats a piece of pie (1/8 of the pie) there will be 7/8 left.

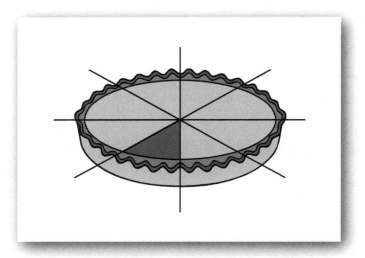

Look at the pie illustration in Figure 3-2. If two families share a pie, and one family eats two pieces while the other eats four, their pie consumption can be expressed as the ratio 2/4 or two to four. This is especially important in pharmacy, where compounding often requires you to think in terms of ratios, or parts per unit.

Figure 3-2. If the Fitz family eats two pieces of the pie, and the Hughes family eats four pieces, the ratio of their pie consumption can be expressed as 2/4 or two to four.

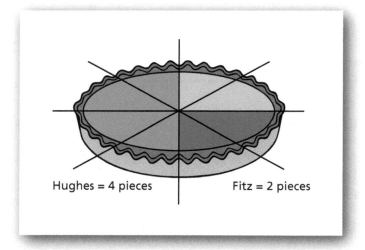

Hughes = 4 pieces   Fitz = 2 pieces

NUMBERS AT WORK
Understanding ratios or fractions is important for compounding medications and preparations.

To simplify a fraction, write the numerator and denominator as products of prime factors. Any factor that is the same in the numerator and in the denominator represents a factor of one and can be cancelled. Remaining factors are then multiplied to yield a simplified fraction.

EXAMPLE

Simplify $\dfrac{8}{50}$

SOLUTION ···

$$\frac{8}{50} = \frac{2 \times 2 \times 2}{2 \times 5 \times 5}$$

$$= \frac{2 \times 2}{5 \times 5}$$

$$= \frac{4}{25}$$

When multiplying fractions, the numerator of the first fraction is multiplied by the numerator of the second fraction and the denominator of the first fraction is multiplied by the denominator of the second fraction. Then the fraction is simplified. To simplify, first write the numerator and denominator as products of prime factors. Any factors that appear in both numerator and denominator can be cancelled before multiplying.

EXAMPLE

Each tablet contains 6/10 of a milligram of colchicine. How many milligrams of colchicine does one half a tablet contain?

SOLUTION ···

$$\frac{1}{2} \times \frac{6}{10}$$

$$= \frac{1 \times 2 \times 3}{2 \times 2 \times 5} = \frac{3}{2 \times 5}$$

$$= \frac{3}{10}$$

So, one half of a tablet contains 3/10 of a milligram of colchicine.

The reciprocal of a fraction is obtained by inverting the original fraction, that is, by interchanging the **numerator** and **denominator**. For example, $\frac{4}{5}$ and $\frac{5}{4}$ are reciprocals. When dividing fractions, multiply the dividend by the reciprocal of the divisor.

Numerator—The portion of a fraction above the fraction line.

Denominator—The part of a fraction that is below the fraction bar, also the divisor of a division problem.

EXAMPLE

One half of a liter (metric measure of volume) of normal saline is to be divided into vials of 1/10 liter each. How many vials are needed?

SOLUTION ....

$$\frac{1}{2} \div \frac{1}{10} = \frac{1}{2} \times \frac{10}{1}$$

$$= \frac{2 \times 5}{2} = 5$$

So, five vials are needed.

To add (or subtract) fractions with the same denominator, add (or subtract) the numerators, place the sum (or difference) over the common denominator and simplify if possible.

EXAMPLE

One container holds 1/10 of a liter of concentrated sodium chloride, another contains 3/10 of a liter. The two solutions are to be combined. Would a ¼ liter or a ½ liter container be needed to hold the solution?

SOLUTION ....

$$\frac{1}{10} + \frac{3}{10}$$

$$= \frac{4}{10} = \frac{2 \times 2}{2 \times 5} = \frac{2}{5}$$

So, a 1/2 liter container is needed, because 2/5 liter is larger than 1/4 liter and less than 1/2 liter.

To add (or subtract) fractions with different denominators, a least common denominator must be calculated. The least common denominator can be calculated in two steps.

1. Write each denominator as the product of prime factors.

2. The least common denominator is the product of a repeated factor times any factors that are not repeated.

EXAMPLE

Find the least common denominator (lcd) of $\frac{2}{3}$, $\frac{1}{6}$, and $\frac{9}{10}$.

SOLUTION ....

3 = 3
6 = 2 × 3 products of prime factors
10 = 2 × 5
2 and 3 are repeated factors, 5 is not.
So the lcd = 2 × 3 × 5 = 30

EXAMPLE

Find the lcd of $\frac{3}{14}$ and $\frac{1}{10}$

SOLUTION ·

$14 = 2 \times 7$
$10 = 2 \times 5$
2 is a repeated factor, 7 and 5 are not.
So, the lcd $= 2 \times 5 \times 7 = 70$

Once the least common denominator is calculated, each fraction is rewritten as an equivalent fraction that has the least common denominator. This is done by multiplying the numerator and denominator by the number that results in the common denominator.

$$\frac{3}{14} \times \frac{5}{5} = \frac{15}{70}$$

$$\frac{1}{10} \times \frac{7}{7} = \frac{7}{70}$$

EXAMPLE

The remains of three containers of Miralax® are to be combined to fill Mrs. Dennison's prescription. They are $\frac{1}{10}$ of a pint, $\frac{2}{5}$ of a pint and $\frac{1}{4}$ of a pint.

How many pints will be in the combined product?

SOLUTION ·

Find the lcd. $\frac{1}{10} + \frac{2}{5} + \frac{1}{4}$

$10 = 2 \times 5$
$5 = 5$
$4 = 2 \times 2$
One factor of 2 is repeated, one factor of 2 is not, and one factor of 5 is repeated.
So, the lcd $= 2 \times 2 \times 5 = 20$

Now, we convert the denominators in each of the original fractions to 20. To accomplish this, multiply each fraction by a fraction equal to one (such as 2/2 or 5/5) so that the new denominator is 20.

$$\frac{1}{10} \times \frac{2}{2} + \frac{2}{5} \times \frac{4}{4} + \frac{1}{4} \times \frac{5}{5}$$

$$= \frac{2 + 8 + 5}{20}$$

$$= \frac{15}{20}$$

$$= \frac{3}{4}$$

So, there is 3/4 of a pint in the finished product.

A mixed number consists of a whole number and a **fraction**. For example, $4\frac{3}{5}$ is a mixed number and is read, "four and three fifths." An **improper fraction** is one in which the numerator is greater than the denominator. To write a mixed number as an improper fraction, multiply the denominator by the whole number. Add this product to the numerator. Place this sum over the denominator.

EXAMPLE

Rewrite $2\frac{5}{7}$ as an improper fraction.

SOLUTION

$7 \times 2 = 14$ multiply denominator by whole number

$14 + 5 = 19$ add product to numerator

$\frac{19}{7}$ place sum over denominator

To write an improper fraction as a mixed number, divide numerator by denominator, and place the remainder over the denominator.

EXAMPLE

Rewrite $\frac{25}{3}$ as a mixed number.

SOLUTION

$$3\overline{)25} \quad \begin{array}{r} 8 \\ \hline \end{array}$$
$$\underline{-24}$$
$$\text{1 remainder}$$

So $\frac{25}{3} = 8\frac{1}{3}$

To multiply or divide two mixed numbers, write each mixed number as an improper fraction, then multiply or divide the resulting fractions.

EXAMPLE

Tylenol® with codeine solution is to be administered in doses of 2½ teaspoonfuls six times per day if needed for pain. How many teaspoonfuls of Tylenol® with codeine may be given in a day?

SOLUTION

$$2\frac{1}{2} \times 6 = \frac{5}{2} \times \frac{6}{1}$$

$$= \frac{30}{2}$$

The result can then be written as a whole number.

$$\frac{30}{2} = 15 \text{ teaspoonfuls}$$

So, 15 teaspoonfuls of Tylenol® with codeine may be given in a day.

EXAMPLE

Find the quotient.

$$3\frac{1}{2} \div 2\frac{1}{3}$$

SOLUTION ··

$$3\frac{1}{2} \div 2\frac{1}{3}$$

$$= \frac{7}{2} \div \frac{7}{3}$$

$$= \frac{7}{2} \times \frac{3}{7}$$

$$= \frac{3}{2}$$

$$= 1\frac{1}{2}$$

To add or subtract mixed numbers, write each as an improper fraction, find the least common denominator, then add or subtract the resulting fractions. The answer can then be written as a mixed number.

EXAMPLE

Dr. Lance Boyle prescribes 2½ teaspoonfuls of docusate liquid and 1¼ teaspoonfuls of Metamucil®. How many teaspoonfuls of medicine are prescribed?

SOLUTION ··

$$2\frac{1}{2} + 1\frac{1}{4} = \frac{5}{2} + \frac{5}{4} \qquad \text{change to improper fractions}$$

$$= \frac{5}{2} \times \frac{2}{2} + \frac{5}{4} \qquad \text{find lcd}$$

$$= \frac{10}{4} + \frac{5}{4}$$

$$= \frac{15}{4} = 3\frac{3}{4} \qquad \text{change to mixed number}$$

So, 3¾ teaspoonfuls of medicine are prescribed.

Decimal fractions

A **decimal fraction** is a fraction in which the denominator is a power of 10 such as 10, 100, or 1000. The denominator of a decimal fraction is not written, but the number of digits to the right of the decimal indicates the place value of the denominator. One digit indicates tenths, two indicates hundredths, three indicates thousandths, four indicates ten thousandths, and so on (see Figure 2-2, in Chapter 2). Any fraction can be written as a decimal fraction by dividing the numerator by the denominator. When using a calculator, make sure to enter the numerator first.

Decimal Fraction—A fraction whose denominator is a power of 10.

EXAMPLE

Write $\frac{1}{8}$ as a decimal fraction.

SOLUTION ·

$$
\begin{array}{r}
0.125 \\
8\overline{)1.000} \\
\underline{-\ 8\ \ } \\
20 \\
\underline{-16\ } \\
40 \\
\underline{-40\ } \\
0
\end{array}
$$

Order of Operations

Mathematical problems are often written out in the form of an equation. An **equation** is a mathematical statement, separated by an equal sign, where each side of the statement is equal. Take a look at the example of an addition problem at the beginning of the chapter, where the two technicians were making IV piggyback bags. When that problem is written as an equation it looks like this:

$$44 \text{ bags} + 27 \text{ bags} = 71 \text{ bags}$$

We can see that $44 + 27$ is another way of expressing the number 71. Thus, each side of an equation is referred to as an expression. All word problems can be written as equations, but sometimes these equations will contain more than one mathematical operation, so it is important to know in what order to perform them.

The rule is that any operation isolated by parentheses is completed first, followed by multiplication and division from the left of the problem to the right and then addition and subtraction from the left to the right.

> **TECH NOTE!**
>
> *Perform math operations in parentheses first, then multiplication and division, from left to right, then addition and subtraction from left to right.*

EXAMPLE

Theresa Jones, R.Ph., is the pharmacist-in-charge for Just Right Pharmacy. She is looking at the cost of buying pharmaceuticals for the past quarter, and wants to determine the average cost per month. Pharmaceuticals cost $19,052.00 in January, $14,363.00 in February, and $22,103.00 in March. What was the average cost/month of pharmaceuticals for the quarter?

SOLUTION ·

Remember that to find an average of a series of numbers, you find the sum of the numbers and then divide by the number of entries in the series.

$$\frac{(\$19{,}052.00 + \$14{,}363.00 + \$22{,}103.00)}{3 \text{ months}} = \$18{,}506/\text{month}$$

Continue to practice and refresh the math skills reviewed in this chapter by completing the practice problems since these skills serve as the foundation for upcoming chapters.

Practice Problems

1. **Find the sum.**
   a. $3 + 9$
   b. $127 + 13$
   c. On Monday, Bill the pharmacist sees 19 customers for prescription consultations and pharmacist Don sees 18 customers for consultations. Altogether, how many customers were seen for consultations on Monday?

2. **Find the difference.**
   a. $18 - 7$
   b. $124 - 39$
   c. The C. F. Eye Care hospital had 100 bottles of artificial tears eye drops on the shelf. Fifty-nine bottles were removed because the expiration date had passed. How many bottles remained on the shelf?

3. **Find the product.**
   a. 8×7
   b. $3 \times 4 \times 14$
   c. Dr. Dee Kay orders that 2 capsules of Zovirax® 200 mg be administered 5 times daily for 14 days. How many capsules are needed?

4. **Find the quotient.**
   a. $100 \div 20$ b. $2\overline{)18}$ c. $\dfrac{14}{6}$

5. **Three hundred vitamin C 250-mg tablets are to be equally distributed among 150 patients.**
   a. How many tablets will each patient receive? Will there be any tablets left over? If so, how many?
   b. One thousand tablets are to be divided into prescription vials containing 30 tablets each. How many vials are needed? Will there be any tablets left over? If so, how many?

6. **Simplify each fraction.**
   a. $\dfrac{3}{12}$ b. $\dfrac{14}{42}$ c. $\dfrac{8}{18}$

7. **Find the product. Write each product in simplest form.**
   a. $\dfrac{2}{9} \times \dfrac{3}{4}$ b. $\dfrac{9}{28} \times \dfrac{14}{27}$ c. $\dfrac{3}{10} \times \dfrac{5}{6}$

8. **Find the quotient. Write each quotient in simplest form.**
   a. $\dfrac{2}{9} \div \dfrac{4}{3}$ b. $\dfrac{9}{10} \div \dfrac{6}{5}$

9. **Find the quotient. Write each quotient in simplest form.**
   a. $\dfrac{2}{27} \div \dfrac{4}{9}$

b. $\dfrac{3}{4}$ of an ounce of hydrocortisone 1% is to be divided into three equal parts. How much will each part contain?

10. **Find the sum or difference. Write each in simplest form.**

    a. $\dfrac{3}{8} + \dfrac{2}{8}$ b. $\dfrac{3}{4} - \dfrac{1}{4}$ c. $\dfrac{1}{9} + \dfrac{2}{9}$ d. $\dfrac{7}{8} - \dfrac{4}{8}$ e. $\dfrac{7}{10} - \dfrac{3}{10}$

11. **Find the sum or difference. Write each in simplest form.**

    a. $\dfrac{2}{3} + \dfrac{1}{4}$ b. $\dfrac{3}{4} + \dfrac{1}{8}$ c. $\dfrac{2}{3} - \dfrac{1}{12}$ d. $\dfrac{2}{9} + \dfrac{5}{12}$ e. $\dfrac{8}{9} - \dfrac{2}{5}$

12. **Rewrite the mixed number as an improper fraction.**

    a. $2\dfrac{3}{4}$ b. $9\dfrac{1}{8}$ c. $4\dfrac{2}{3}$

13. **Rewrite the improper fraction as a mixed number.**

    a. $\dfrac{14}{3}$ b. $\dfrac{21}{5}$ c. $\dfrac{14}{9}$

14. **Find the product.**

    a. $2\dfrac{1}{3} \times \dfrac{3}{4}$ b. $4\dfrac{1}{2} \times 1\dfrac{1}{9}$ c. $2\dfrac{2}{3} \times 1\dfrac{1}{4}$

15. **Find the quotient.**

    a. $6\dfrac{2}{3} \div \dfrac{5}{3}$

    b. $3\dfrac{1}{2}$ ounces of Robitussin DM® is to be divided into portions that are $\dfrac{1}{4}$ ounce each. How many portions will there be?

    c. $2\dfrac{1}{2}$ tsp of amoxicillin suspension is to be given in two equal doses. How many tsp will there be in each dose?

16. **Find the sum.**

    a. $3\dfrac{1}{6} + 1\dfrac{5}{8}$

    b. Baby George is to be given 2½ teaspoonfuls of prednisone 1 mg/mL each morning and 1¼ teaspoonfuls in the afternoon. How many teaspoonfuls of prednisone are to be taken each day?

17. **Rewrite the fraction as a decimal fraction.**

    a. $\dfrac{3}{8}$ b. $\dfrac{9}{10}$ c. $\dfrac{4}{5}$

18. **Dr. Denton prescribes one tablet of pseudoephedrine 60 mg to be taken twice daily for 1 month for patient Constance Noring. How many tablets should be dispensed?**

19. **Dr. Gohan N. Sumi directs patient Nora Maki to take one capsule of Augmentin® 250 mg three times a day for 14 days. How many capsules should be dispensed?**

20. Mrs. Johnson is asked to give her daughter Pam ¾ teaspoonful of Bactrim® Suspension 2 times a day for 14 days. The pharmacist fills the order with a bottle of 20 tsp. Is this enough to last for 30 days?

21. Wanda Hu gets three prescriptions filled every month. Although her insurance company provides prescription coverage, she pays a co-pay for each prescription. For her birth control tablets she pays $15.00, for her albuterol inhaler she pays $15.00, but for her Advair® inhaler she pays $65.00 each month. What is the average co-pay Wanda pays?

22. At the class picnic hot dog eating contest, the senior class representative eats 12 hot dogs in 15 minutes, while the junior class contestant can only manage 8 hot dogs in 15 minutes.
    a. Write each class's hot dog eating results as a ratio of hot dogs/time, and reduce each to hot dogs per minute.
    b. Which class won the contest?

23. Nat Faste, the representative from Code Blue Insurance Company, has granted approval for Wright Pharmacy to fill a 90-day supply of Evan Tooly's prescription. He takes two ibuprofen 400-mg tablets three times daily. How many tablets does Nat need to fill this prescription?

24. Complete the table.

Fraction	Decimal	Percent
1/2	0.5	50%
	0.375	37.5%
3/4		75%
	0.80	80%
	0.25	25%
2/5		40%

25. The pharmacist asks the pharmacy technician to divide 2000 grams of zinc oxide ointment into several sized jars. He would like the technician to fill ten 60-gram jars, eleven 90-gram jars, and six 30-gram jars.
    a. What is the total amount of zinc oxide used to fill all the jars?
    b. Write the ratio of the amount in the 60-gram jars over the total amount of zinc oxide ointment used and reduce to the simplest form.
    c. Write the fraction determined in Part b as a decimal.

Systems of Measurement

CHAPTER 4

The Metric System

LEARNING OBJECTIVES

1. Identify prefixes and abbreviations used in the metric system.
2. Convert between units within the metric system.
3. Add and subtract quantities expressed with metric units.
4. List the basic units of measurement in the metric system and identify a familiar object or length that approximates each unit.
5. Use dimensional analysis to solve conversion problems.

Introduction

The **metric system** of measurement is a decimal system, like our money, based on powers of ten. Common prefixes for powers of ten, their meanings and abbreviations are shown in Table 4-1. This system is the international standard for measurements. In the United States, the metric system is used in research, university, health care and most governmental settings, but we have been slow to adopt it in our homes. As you become more familiar with this system, you will discover it is actually easier to use than our current household system.

Metric System—The decimal measuring system based on the meter, liter, and gram as units of length, capacity, and weight or mass.

Table 4-1. Metric Unit Prefix, Meaning, and Abbreviation

Prefix	Meaning	Abbreviation
kilo	1000	k
deci	1/10 = 0.1	d
centi	1/100 = 0.01	c
milli	1/1000 = 0.001	m
micro	1/1,000,000 = 0.000001	mc

Metric Measurements

There are three basic units of measurement in the metric system: the **meter**, which measures length, the **gram**, which measures mass (commonly thought of as weight) and the **liter**, which measures volume.

Length

The metric system was devised to standardize measurements used for international trade. The meter was first established in France in 1798 as one ten-millionth of the distance from the equator to the North Pole. Today 1 meter is defined as

Meter—The standard unit of length in the metric system.

Gram—Standard unit of mass in the metric system.

Liter—Standard unit of volume in the metric system.

the distance light travels in a vacuum in 1/299,792,548 of a second. While this definition is quite precise, it may not be too meaningful to most of us. As a rule of thumb, 1 meter is about the distance that most doorknobs are from the floor. It is also easy to remember that for the average sized man, the distance from his nose, across the shoulder to the tip of his outstretched hand is about 1 meter (see Figure 4-1). The abbreviation for meter is m.

Figure 4-1. A meter is approximately the distance from a man's nose to the tip of his outstretched hand.

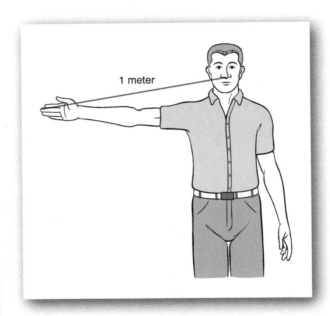

Weight

One gram is the weight of a cube of water that is one centimeter (1 cm) on each side in the refrigerator at sea level. The abbreviation for gram is g. A nickel weighs 5 grams, and a dollar bill or a business card weighs approximately 1 gram (see Figure 4-2). Medicine is often weighed in thousandths of a gram, called a milligram, abbreviated mg and in millionths of a gram called a microgram, abbreviated mcg.

Volume

One liter is the volume of 1000 cubes that are all one centimeter on each side, and is abbreviated as L. Most of us are familiar with a 2-liter bottle soft drink. To get an idea of what 1 liter looks like, a quart is just short of a liter (see Figure 4-2). In the pharmacy, liquids are often measured in thousandths of liters or milliliters, abbreviated mL. One milliliter is the volume of one cubic centimeter of refrigerated water at sea level. In some fields the abbreviation cc (cubic centimeter) is used interchangeably with mL. However, in health care, the abbreviation cc can be misinterpreted, so when referring to volume measurements we use only milliliters, or mL.

Figure 4-2. Common objects that approximate metric units.

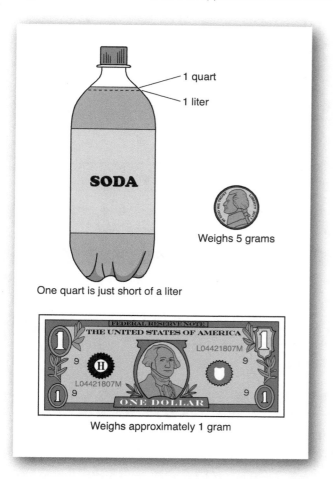

1 quart

1 liter

SODA

Weighs 5 grams

One quart is just short of a liter

Weighs approximately 1 gram

NUMBERS AT WORK

In pharmacy, 1/1000 of a liter is designated as a milliliter or mL. The term "cc" is not used.

Conversions Within the Metric System

For conversions within the metric system, multiply or divide by a power of 10, which is the same as moving the decimal place in the original measurement. When making conversions, first ask, "Is the new unit larger or smaller than the original unit?" If the new unit is smaller than the original unit, then multiply, or move the decimal to the right, in order to convert. For example, if you want to convert grams to milligrams, multiply grams by 1000 (see Figure 4-3).

If the new unit is larger than the original unit, divide, or move the decimal to the left to convert to the larger unit.

Figure 4-3. The movement of the decimal point for metric conversions.

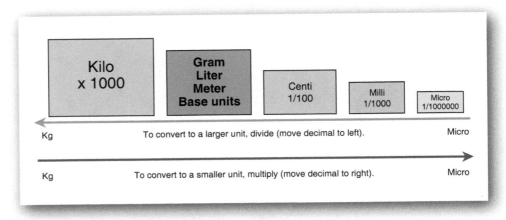

EXAMPLE

If 10 mL contains 2 grams of cefazolin, how many milligrams are in the same volume?

SOLUTION ···

1 gram = 1000 milligrams. One mg is a smaller unit than 1 g, so multiply grams by 1000 to convert to mg.

2 g̶ × 1000 mg/g̶ = 2000 mg

If the new unit is larger than the original unit, then you will divide by a power of 10 to convert between the two.

EXAMPLE

Convert 2340 mg to g

SOLUTION ···

The new units (grams) are larger than the original units (milligrams), so divide to convert. One gram is 1000 mg, so divide by 1000, or move the decimal point three places to the left.

2340 mg = 2.340 g

EXAMPLE

Convert 0.256 L to mL

SOLUTION ···

The new units (milliliters) are smaller than the original units (liters). A liter is 1000 milliliters, so multiply by 1000, or move the decimal point three places to the right.

0.256 L = 256 mL

EXAMPLE

Convert 5,250 mcg to mg

SOLUTION ···

The new units (milligrams) are larger than the original units (micrograms). One microgram is 1/1000 or 0.001 of a milligram, so divide by 1000, or move the decimal point three places to the left.

5250 mcg = 5.25 mg

EXAMPLE

Convert 5,678.911 mg to g

SOLUTION ···

The new units (grams) are larger than the original units (milligrams). One milligram is 1/1000 or 0.001 of a gram, so move the decimal point three places to the left.

5,678.911 mg = 5.678911 g, which can be rounded to 5.7 g

It is sometimes necessary to add or subtract metric measurements. For example, it may be important to calculate the total dose of a medication taken by a patient during a day. In order to do such a calculation, the units of the numbers must all be the same.

> **TECH NOTE!**

When adding or subtracting measurements, all quantities must have the same units.

EXAMPLE

Add 0.25 L + 375 mL

SOLUTION ···

First convert mL to L by dividing by 1,000, or move the decimal point three places to the left.

375 mL = 0.375 L
0.25 L + 0.375 L = 0.625 L
= 625 mL

> **EXAMPLE**
>
> Subtract 576 mg – 432 mcg
>
> **SOLUTION** ··
>
> 576 mg = 576,000 mcg
> 576,000 mcg – 432 mcg = 575,568 mcg
> To convert mcg to mg, divide by 1000 or move the decimal point three places
> to the right.
> = 575.568 mg

Using dimensional analysis

Dimensional analysis is a technique for converting between units. When applying dimensional analysis, multiply by a conversion factor or ratio whose value is 1. For example, 1 g/1000 mg is such a ratio because 1 gram is the equivalent of 1000 mg. Use a conversion chart and the problem to choose an equivalency. First, look at the problem to determine the desired units for the answer. Next, choose an equivalency that relates the given units to the desired units. Now, the equivalency is stated as a ratio, or fraction. The hardest part is deciding which way the ratio should be written. For example, the relationship between grams and mg may be written as:

$$1 \text{ g}/1000 \text{ mg}$$
or as:
$$1000 \text{ mg}/\text{g}$$

The ratio you choose must have the desired units (for the answer) in the numerator. After you work the problem, if the units don't cancel out to what is needed, you will know that you have worked the problem incorrectly.

> ▶ *TECH NOTE!*
>
> *When using dimensional analysis, the units must cancel out to the*
> *units desired in the answer.*

Table 4-2. Common Metric Conversions

Metric units of weight

1 kg	1000 g	1,000,000 mg	1,000,000,000 mcg
	1 g	1000 mg	1,000,000 mcg
		1 mg	1000 mcg

Metric units of volume

1 L	10 dL	100 cL	1000 mL

Metric units of length

1 km	1000 m	100,000 cm	1,000,000 mm
	1 m	100 cm	1000 mm

EXAMPLE

Convert 385 mg to grams

SOLUTION ··

From Table 4-2, we see that 1 g = 1000 mg
Divide both sides of this equation by 1000 mg to obtain a ratio equal to one
that contains the desired units.

$$\frac{1\ g}{1000\ mg} = 1$$

So:

$$385\ mg\ (1) = 385\ mg\left(\frac{1\ g}{1000\ mg}\right) = 0.385\ g$$

EXAMPLE

Convert 0.75 L to mL.

SOLUTION ··

From Table 4-2, determine that 1000 mL = 1 L
Divide both sides of this equation by 1 liter to obtain a ratio that contains
the desired units.

$$\frac{1000\ mL}{L} = 1$$

So, $0.75\ L\ (1) = 0.75\ L\left(\dfrac{1000\ mL}{L}\right) = 750\ mL$

Practice Problems

Choose the most appropriate metric unit of weight, volume, or length for the following problems. Choose from the following options: m, cm, mm, L, mL, g, kg, or mg.

1. Medication directions call for 5 _____ of cough syrup to be given to a child.

2. One dime weighs about 2 _____.

3. Soda is sold in bottles containing 2 _____.

4. A pet cat weighs 4 _____.

5. A letter weighs about 20–30 _____.

6. John is about 200 _____ tall.

7. Directions call for 500 _____ of vitamin C to be taken daily.

8. Orders call for 0.1 _____ of tuberculin solution to be injected under the skin for a TB skin test.

9. Rewrite, using a numeral and the appropriate abbreviation.
   a. One hundred fifty milliliters
   b. Thirty-four micrograms
   c. Sixty-five liters
   d. Three hundred thirty milligrams
   e. Nine hundred fifty-five grams
   f. Five kilograms

10. Rewrite in words.
    a. 915 mcg
    b. 30 L
    c. 145 mL
    d. 160 mg
    e. 175 g
    f. 10 kg

11. Make the following conversions.
    a. 150 mcg to milligrams
    b. 2000 mL to liters
    c. 845 kg to grams
    d. 1.575 g to kilograms
    e. 3000 mg to grams
    f. 5000 mg to micrograms
    g. 5.35 L to milliliters
    h. 1775 kg to grams
    i. 350 mcg to grams
    j. 14.567 g to milligrams

12. **Rewrite, using a decimal number and the appropriate abbreviation.**
    a. five tenths of a gram
    b. three tenths of a milligram
    c. five and two tenths of a gram
    d. three hundredths of a liter
    e. five and six tenths of a milliliter

13. **Add 300 mL + 4 L + 1.5 L. Express answer in milliliters and in liters.**

14. **Add 5000 mg + 7 g. Express answer in milligrams and in grams.**

15. **Add 455 mg + 365 mcg. Express answer in milligrams and in micrograms.**

16. **Subtract: 2 L – 500 mL. Express answer in liters and milliliters.**

17. **Subtract: 3 g – 3 mg. Express answer in grams and milligrams.**

18. **Subtract: 2.5 mg – 100 mcg. Express answer in milligrams and micrograms.**

19. **Subtract: 2.5 L – 1.2 L. Express answer in liters and milliliters.**

20. **Subtract: 1 L – 750 mL. Express answer in liters and milliliters.**

21. **Choose the appropriate conversion factor to convert milligrams to grams.**

22. **Choose the appropriate conversion factor to convert grams to milligrams.**

23. **Choose the appropriate conversion factor(s) to convert mcg to kg.**

24. **Use dimensional analysis to make the following conversions:**
    a. 1.5 kg = _____ mg
    b. 30 mL = _____ L
    c. 5.1 km = _____ cm
    d. 175,000 mcg = _____ kg

25. **Anita DeSmall, Ph.T., receives a prescription for levothyroxine 0.125-mg tablets. She fills the prescription with levothyroxine 125-mcg tablets. Use dimensional analysis to determine if Anita dispensed the correct drug.**

CHAPTER 5

Apothecary and Household Measurements and Metric Conversions

LEARNING OBJECTIVES

1. List the metric equivalents of 1 fluid ounce, 1 tablespoonful, and 1 teaspoonful.
2. List the metric equivalent of 1 pound, 1 ounce, and 1 grain.
3. Convert a patient's weight in pounds to kilograms, or in kilograms to pounds.
4. Explain why it is important for technicians to be completely comfortable using and converting to the metric system.
5. Use dimensional analysis to convert between units.

Introduction

In the period of time during and after the Renaissance, the study of science and medicine began in earnest. At that point in history there was no consistent, international system of weights and measures. Measurements of mass (usually referred to as weight) were based on commonly weighed materials, such as a grain of wheat or a penny. Different systems of measurements were used for different applications. For example, people who worked in the trades used a different system of measurement than jewelers or apothecaries.

The **apothecary** was a member of the healing arts who was the predecessor of today's pharmacist and a specialist in the preparation of medicines and remedies. Apothecaries dispensed remedies, performed surgery, or assisted in childbirth. In order to prepare the remedies consistently, apothecaries needed a systematic method for weighing and measuring ingredients.

Apothecary System of Weights and Measures

Apothecary units

The **apothecary system** of weights and measures was related to the Roman system of measurement. This system is based on the grain (abbreviated gr) as a measurement of weight, and the fluid ounce (fl oz) as a measurement of volume. There are some similarities between apothecary measurements, common household, and **avoirdupois** measurements (the system of weights and measures historically used in the U.S. and Great Britain), but also some significant differences. The apothecary pound, for instance, is divided into 12 ounces, but the avoirdupois pound is divided into 16 ounces. The dry ounce is a measure of weight. To avoid confusion, you will learn conversions for ounces and pounds from the household and avoirdupois system of measurement only.

Apothecary—A member of the healing arts who was the predecessor of today's pharmacists.

Apothecary System—This system is based on the grain as a measurement of weight, and the fluid ounce as a measurement of volume.

Avoirdupois System—The system of weights and measures historically used in the U.S. and Great Britain.

The minim, fluid dram (fl dr), and fluid ounce are the measurements of volume in the apothecary system. The word "fluid" indicates a measure of volume. Where the apothecary system is used to measure volume, symbols may represent these units. Table 5-1 shows the conversion factors and symbols in the apothecary system.

Table 5-1. Most Likely Measurements a Technician Will Encounter

pint	fl ounce	fl dram
1 pt	16 fl oz	128 fl dram
	1 fl oz	8 fl dram
		1 fl dram

Pt = pint, fl = fluid.

Although the apothecary system of measurement was the standard for the practice of pharmacy into the 20th century in the United States, it was officially replaced by the metric system in 1971. Use of apothecary measurements is discouraged because they are less user-friendly than the metric system, and they are not universally recognized. It is not unheard of, however, for older physicians to write prescriptions using the apothecary system. To be adequately prepared for work in a variety of pharmacy practice settings, students need to be familiar with the more common of the apothecary measurements.

Household and Avoirdupois Weights and Measures

Units of weight and volume

Most people who have followed a recipe at home or prepared boxed dinners or desserts are familiar with the household system of measurement. Household measurements of weight (mass) are based on the avoirdupois system, which, like the apothecary system is an antiquated system of measurement. The avoirdupois system is only used to measure weight, and the basic unit is the ounce (oz). Household measurements of volume include the teaspoon (abbreviated tsp), tablespoon (abbreviated T), fluid ounce, cup (c), pint (pt), quart (qt), and gallon (gal). See Table 5-2.

Table 5-2. Common Household Measurements of Volume and Weight

Measurements of Volume

1 gallon	4 quarts	8 pints	16 cups	128 fl oz	256 tablesponful (T)	768 tsp
	1 quart	2 pints	4 cups	32 fl oz	64 T	192 tsp
		1 pint	2 cups	16 fl oz	32 T	96 tsp
			1 cup	8 fl oz	16 T	48 tsp
				1 fl oz	2 T	6 tsp
					1 T	3 tsp

Measurements of Weight

1 pound	16 ounces

Measuring doses accurately

Doses of liquid medications in outpatient prescriptions are often written as teaspoons or tablespoons because these measurements are more familiar to American patients than metric units. The problem with directions of this type is that household teaspoons and tablespoons vary widely in the actual volume they hold (see Figure 5-1). The volume of a teaspoon, for instance, can range from 4 to 7 mL. This difference means that a person trying to measure a 5 mL (one teaspoonful) dose could get a dose that ranged from 20% less to 40% more than desired. This is unacceptable for measuring medications, especially for children, where a dose variation of this magnitude can be dangerous.

Figure 5-1. Volume variations in common household teaspoons.

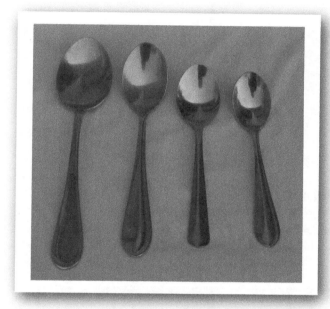

To prevent inaccuracy of dosing measurements, it is important that patients have appropriate measuring devices in their homes, and are instructed in how to use them. Choosing the correct device to measure volume depends on the age of the patient. Infants will do better taking medication from a **calibrated** (marked with measurement lines) oral syringe or dropper, while toddlers are able to use a dosing spoon (see Figure 5-2). Adults taking liquid medications can use a calibrated medicine cup. These devices are labeled with both household and metric measurements. In retail or other outpatient pharmacies, it is good practice to include both metric and household measurements in the directions on a prescription label for a liquid medication.

Calibrated—Marked with measurement lines.

Figure 5-2. Medication can be measured with calibrated droppers, cups, oral syringes, or dosing spoons.

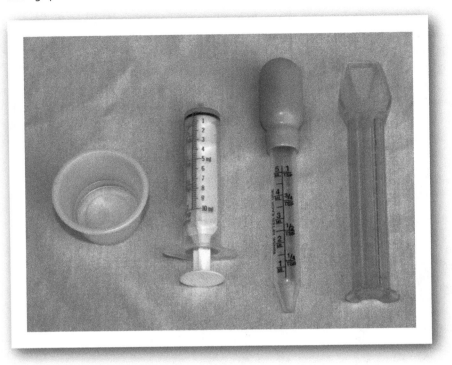

NUMBERS AT WORK

In retail or other outpatient pharmacies, it is good practice to include both metric and household measurements in the directions on a prescription label for a liquid medication.

EXAMPLE

What would be the clearest way to write the directions for the following prescription?

Max Price, MD
1349 Beverly Drive
Beverly Hills, CA (213) 555-5505

Name: Golda Barr   Date: 11/10

Address: _____

Rx   Donnatal Elixir 120 mL

    5 mL Q 8 h prn stomach upset

refill 0 ① 2 3
dea # am123456   _____Max Price_____ MD

SOLUTION ··

Bell's Drug Store
522 E. Veterans Ave, Los Angeles, CA
Tel: 555-5405

Rx: 123456   Date: 6/30/12
Golda Barr
Take one teaspoonful (5 ml) every eight hours if needed for stomach upset

Donnatal Liquid (clear green soln) 120 mL
Exp: 6/30/2012

Working problems using household measurements

There are times when you may need to solve problems and use conversion factors within the household system. If you are a cook, you may already know how to make these conversions. When solving problems that require a conversion, it helps to begin by converting the units in the problem to whatever unit is necessary for the answer.

> **TECH NOTE!**
>
> *The first step in solving conversion problems: make the necessary conversions for measurements in the problem to the units needed for the answer.*

EXAMPLE

The pharmacy technician at Best Rx Pharmacy received a prescription for 16 fluid ounces of Robitussin AC®. She opened a new gallon bottle earlier that morning and filled three other prescriptions, one for a pint of Robitussin AC® and two for 6 fluid ounces each. How many fluid ounces of Robitussin AC will be left after she fills the new prescription?

SOLUTION ··

Step 1. Convert 1 gallon and one pint to fluid ounces (see Table 5-2).
          1 gallon = 128 fl oz
          1 pint = 16 fl oz

Step 2. Add up the total volume dispensed in fluid ounces.
          16 fl oz + 6 fl oz + 6 fl oz + 16 fl oz = 44 fl oz dispensed

Step 3. Find the difference between the volume in the original container and the amount dispensed to determine the fluid ounces remaining.
          128 fl oz – 44 fl oz = 84 fl oz remaining

Occasionally problems produce answers expressed in something other than units of measurement. In the following problem you will still need to make a conversion, but the final answer will be expressed in total items, rather than units of measurement.

EXAMPLE

Pharmacist Bea Blessing needs to restock the nursery unit with zinc oxide ointment, but the 1.5-ounce tubes are unavailable from the manufacturer. She asks new pharmacy technician Sol Smart to transfer one pound of 10% zinc oxide ointment into as many 1.5-ounce jars as he can make. How many jars will Sol need?

SOLUTION ···

Step 1. Convert one pound to ounces. There are 16 ounces in 1 pound.
Step 2. Divide 16 ounces into 1.5 ounce parts to determine how many jars Sol can fill.

$$\frac{16 \text{ oz}}{1.5 \text{ oz per jar}} = 10.7 \text{ jars}$$

Step 3. Look at your answer and see if it makes sense. When a question asks for a whole number of items, an answer with a fraction or a remainder will not work. In this case, Sol will be able to fill only ten jars to the required volume.

Converting Between Systems of Measurement

While the average American knows what a quart is, and may know that there are 8 ounces in a cup, most people around the world are unfamiliar with these units of measurement. A European or Asian cook would be hard pressed to figure out an American recipe, because other countries use the metric system. In this country we use household measures at home, and the metric system in laboratories, hospitals, and universities.

Learning the equivalents for weight and volume measurements across different systems is essential for pharmacy technicians. Like learning times tables, learning conversions is something that requires memorization of the basic relationships. Once these basic conversions are memorized, you will be better able to visualize the relationship between metric, household, and apothecary units of measurement. For example, most of us can picture what a one pound box of powdered sugar looks like and can imagine what it feels like in our hands. Chances are good that most people can identify a 16-ounce beverage, as well. Very few Americans associate that same one pound box or 16-ounce bottle with its equivalent weight in grams, or volume in milliliters (see Figure 5-3).

When you can visualize what 5 grams or 500 milliliters look like, that will allow you to better estimate answers to conversion problems. Developing a feel for conversions and becoming a practiced estimator will improve the odds of identifying wrong answers when making a calculation, a skill that is extremely important for assuring patient safety.

NUMBERS AT WORK
Visualizing the relationship between different units of measure such as liters and gallons can help the technician note potential errors during calculations.

Figure 5-3. Image comparing pint bottle, quart, liter, pound, and kg.

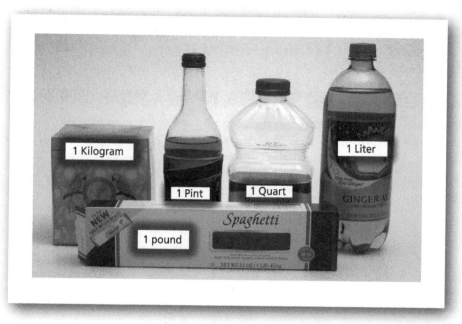

Conversion factors

Table 5-3 shows the conversions from household and apothecary systems to the metric system and back again. The conversion factors listed are rounded from the exact conversions for easier calculations. Some references round conversion factors even further, but at the risk of greater inaccuracy. For example, some calculations textbooks equate 1 liter with 1 quart, and one grain with 60 mg. This comparison is useful for estimating, but is too inaccurate for pharmacy compounding.

Table 5-3. Common Metric, Household, and Apothecary Conversion Factors

Metric Measurement	Household Measurement	Apothecary Measurement
0.065 g (65 mg)[a]		1 grain (gr)
1 g		15.4 gr
28.4 g	1 ounce (oz)	
0.454 kg (454 g)	1 pound (lb)	
1 kg	2.2 lb	
1 L	1.06 quart	
948 mL (960 mL)	1 quart	
474 mL (480 mL)	1 pint	
237 mL (240 mL)	1 cup (8 fl oz)	
29.6 mL (30 mL)	1 fl oz	8 fl drams
15 mL	1 tablespoonful (T)	
5 mL	1 teaspoonful (tsp)	
4 mL		1 fluid dram = 60 minims

[a]Numbers in parentheses reflect 30 mL = 1 fluid ounce.

Problems that require conversions between systems

When working conversion problems between systems of measurement the same rules apply as when converting within one system of measurement. Be extra careful keeping track of units. Consider the problem of converting a patient's weight in pounds to kilograms, below.

EXAMPLE

Baby Mari Noell was admitted to the hospital for suspected meningitis. The orders for Mari read: Ceftriaxone 40 mg/kg IV every 12 hours to start now. How much ceftriaxone will Mari receive in each dose? Baby Mari weighs 32 pounds.

SOLUTION

Step 1. Convert Mari's weight to kg.

$$\frac{32\ lb}{2.2\ lb/kg} = 14.5\ kg$$

As you can see in the solution, by dividing pounds by pounds, these units cancel and the answer will be in kilograms.

Step 2. Calculate the dose of ceftriaxone Mari will receive.

$$40\ mg/kg \times 14.5\ kg = 580\ mg$$

In most pharmacy practice settings, depending on policy, this dose would be rounded to 600 mg of ceftriaxone so that the measurement of the dose is accurate and reproducible.

Once again, in the problem above, all the units except milligrams cancel out. Cancelling units is a good way to check that the equation is set up properly. If you end up with units at the end of a calculation that are not the desired units, the equation was probably set up incorrectly.

For example, when converting pounds to kilograms it is not uncommon for technician students to end up with a weight that is a larger number than the weight expressed in pounds. This usually means that the student lost track of the units and multiplied the number of pounds by 2.2 pounds/kg instead of dividing it. If this were an actual dosing calculation, the result would be that the patient would receive a 4.8-fold dosing error. If units are tracked, this kind of error is prevented. Look at the problem below to understand how you would correctly solve this type of conversion. Remember that a patient's weight expressed in pounds will always be a higher number than his or her weight expressed as kilograms.

> ▶ **TECH NOTE!**
>
> *A patient's weight expressed as pounds will always be a higher number than his or her weight expressed as kilograms.*

EXAMPLE

Juan Ramirez brings in a prescription for son Jaime, who has an ear infection. He notices his 10-month-old son's weight is written as 9.4 kilograms on the prescription, but he would like to be able to tell his wife how much Jaime weighs in pounds. You offer to calculate the weight for him.

SOLUTION ··

Notice that there are two conversion factors that can be used for this problem. First, decide what conversion factor you will use. You can either multiply Jaime's weight in kg by 2.2 pounds/kg, or you can divide his weight by 0.454 kg/pound (see Table 5-3). Try both methods to verify that you get the same answer.

Convert using 2.2 lb/kg: 9.4 kg x 2.2 lb/kg = 20.7 lb

or

convert using 0.454 kg/lb: $\dfrac{9.4\ kg}{0.454\ kg/lb} = 20.7\ lb$

The problem above illustrates an important point. Whether taking a test, or working in the pharmacy, remember that there may be more than one way to solve conversion problems and come out with the correct answer. While you may not always remember all conversion factors, it may be possible to remember enough to solve the problem. Look at one more example to illustrate this concept.

EXAMPLE

Crystal Ball is a new pharmacy technician in the midst of taking the pharmacy technician certification exam. She is asked to calculate the number of tablespoons in a 90-mL bottle. In the stress of the moment, she cannot seem to remember that one tablespoon is 15 mL, but she does remember that 1 ounce is 30 mL and that there are 6 teaspoons per fluid ounce and 3 teaspoons per tablespoon. Can she solve this problem?

SOLUTION ··

Yes, she can. First, she will calculate the number of fluid ounces in 90 mL.

$$\frac{90\ mL}{30\ mL/fl\ oz} = 3\ fl\ oz$$

Next, she will determine the number of teaspoons in 3 fluid ounces.

$$3\ fl\ oz \times 6\ tsp/fl\ oz = 18\ tsp$$

Now, because she remembers there are 3 teaspoons in 1 tablespoon, she can finish the problem.

$$18\ tsp \times \frac{1\ T}{3\ tsp} = 6\ T$$

The best way to assure that you will be able to accurately solve problems that involve conversions is to memorize the conversions and practice the problems. Just as important, if you keep track of a problem's units and learn to estimate before you calculate, you may be able to avoid serious errors by recognizing answers that do not make sense.

▶ *TECH NOTE!* ─────────────────────────

Always estimate before you calculate to reduce the risk of serious errors.

Practice Problems

1. Convert the following to milligrams:
   a. 5 grain = _____ mg
   b. 1.25 grain = _____ mg
   c. 1/150 grain = _____ mg
   d. 10 grain = _____ mg

2. Convert to mg:
   a. 0.1 oz = _____mg
   b. 1/8 grain = _____mg

3. Convert to the units indicated in the first blank, then use that answer to complete the second conversion in each problem below.
   a. 15 mL = _____ fl oz = _____tsp
   b. 1 pint = _____ mL = _____ L
   c. ½ pint = _____ quart = _____ L
   d. 0.25 L = _____mL = _____ fl oz

4. Convert the following to grams:
   a. 0.5 ounce = _____ g
   b. 3/8 pound = _____ g
   c. 1.5 oz = _____ g
   d. ¾ grain = _____ g

5. Number the following in order from 1–6, smallest to largest volume:
   a. liter   _____
   b. fl oz   _____
   c. tablespoon   _____
   d. mL   _____
   e. pint   _____
   f. quart   _____

6. Convert the following to milliliters:
   a. 2 fl drams
   b. 4 fl oz
   c. 2 quarts
   d. 12 fl oz

7. Convert the following as indicated in the problem:
   a. 1.25 L = _____ quart
   b. 8 fl oz = _____ mL
   c. 20 mL = _____ tsp
   d. 180 mL = _____ fl oz

8. Number the following weights in order from smallest to largest, 1–6:
   a. 10,000 mcg _____
   b. 1 mg _____
   c. 5 grain _____

    d. 0.9 g _____

    e. 1 oz _____

    f. ½ lb _____

9. **Change the following to milligrams:**

    a. 0.4 lb

    b. 1.1 kg

    c. 8 ounces

    d. 20 grains

10. **Convert the following body weights as indicated in the problem:**

    a. Newborn: 10.3 pounds = _____ kg

    b. 1 year old: 21 pounds = _____ kg

    c. 5 year old: 21.8 kg = _____ lb

    d. 18 year old: 77.6 kg = _____ lb

    e. 26 year old: 135 pounds = _____ kg

    f. 35 year old: 264.5 pounds = _____ kg

In problems 11–14, match the "drug orders" to the correct metric dosage strengths in the list below. (Note*: some pharmaceutical companies equate 60 mg with 1 grain.)

11. **Thyroid extract 2 grains PO daily**

12. **Acetaminophen 10 gr supp PR q 4 h prn temp >101**

13. **Nitroglycerin 1/200 gr SL tab prn chest pain**

14. **Aspirin 1¼ grain PO daily**

    a. Thyroid 30 mg

    b. Nitroglycerin 0.4 mg SL tab

    c. Aspirin 325 mg

    d. Acetaminophen 650 mg supp

    e. Chewable aspirin 81 mg

    f. Thyroid 120 mg

    g. Acetaminophen 120 mg supp

    h. Nitroglycerin 0.3 mg

15. **Round the conversion factors found in Table 5-3 and the measurements in the problems to check (estimate) whether the following answers are correct. If you believe the answers given are incorrect, explain how you think the error was made.**

    a. Baby John Doe weighs 4 pounds 6 ounces. Odessa Baddun, the technician, receives a drug order for 0.2 mg/kg indomethacin PO x 1 dose. She calculates the dose as 4 mg indomethacin.
    Correct or incorrect?

    b. You are filling a prescription for crotamiton lotion to treat the entire Peste family for scabies. After bathing, each family member is to apply lotion to the body. They are to repeat this procedure the next day, then shower to remove the lotion the following day. The pharmacist thinks 30 mL should be adequate for each application for the children and 60 mL for the adults. There are two adults and 4 children. The pharmacist calculates that ½ pint total of the lotion is adequate for both treatments for the whole family.

Correct or incorrect?

16. Sara James is a 34-year-old female with an acute infection of the kidneys. The hospital-based physician orders tobramycin 2 mg/kg as a one-time loading dose, and requests pharmacist-managed dosing after that. The pharmacist asks you to calculate the first dose. Sara weighs 145 pounds.

   a. What is Sara's weight in kg?

   b. How much tobramycin will Sara receive in the first dose (rounded to the nearest 10 mg)?

   c. Tobramycin solution contains 40 mg tobramycin in 1 mL. How much tobramycin solution is required to make the dose calculated in Part b?

17. The technician at SuperRx Pharmacy receives a new prescription from Mrs. Moody and checks the electronic patient profile to verify the patient information is complete. Technicians at the pharmacy usually get the weight from the patient in pounds and calculate the weight in kilograms. The record indicates Mrs. Moody weighs 113 pounds, or 249 kg. What is wrong with this information and how do you think the error occurred?

For problems 18–20, calculate the amount required per the drug orders.

18. Amoxicillin 20 mg/kg/dose is ordered for James Town. James is 3 years old and weighs 30 pounds. How much amoxicillin per dose will he receive?

19. The veterinarian ordered furosemide 2 mg/kg twice a day for Les Waters' dog, which has heart failure. Round the weight to the nearest kg.

   a. His dog weighs 45 pounds. How much will the dog receive in one dose?

   b. Les' prescription indicates the furosemide solution contains 10 mg/mL. What volume will he measure for one dose?

20. April Schauer has a fever. Her mother states that the pediatrician ordered acetaminophen 20 mg/kg of body weight for her first dose, and then acetaminophen 15 mg/kg every 6 hours after that while her oral temperature is 100° F or more. April weighs 66 pounds.

   a. How much acetaminophen should April's mother give her for the first dose?

   b. What should April's subsequent acetaminophen doses be?

21. A physician orders nitroglycerin 1/150 grain to be placed under the tongue for chest pain. The pharmacy carries nitroglycerin 0.4 mg and nitroglycerin 0.6 mg. Which is correct for this order? (Note: Pharmaceutical companies that make nitroglycerin assume 60 mg = 1 grain.)

22. Convert the following measurements as indicated:

   a. 1 tablespoon = _____ mL   c. 2.5 L = _____ pint

   b. 1 teaspoon = _____ mL   d. 500 mL = _____ fl oz

23. In 1 week during flu season, the pharmacy where you work received six different prescriptions for Hycodan® cough syrup. These include two prescriptions for 4 fl oz, one prescription for 240 mL, one prescription for 180 mL, one prescription for 120 mL, and one prescription for 6 fl oz.

   a. What is the total number of fl oz of Hycodan® dispensed that week?

   b. How many mL of Hycodan® were dispensed that week?

24. A full bottle of nitroglycerin 0.6 mg contains 25 sublingual tablets. How many grains of nitroglycerin are in a full bottle?

25. Dr. Ole Mann still orders acetaminophen with codeine the old-fashioned way. Using the conversion formula provided in this text, how many milligrams of codeine should be in each tablet of the strengths listed below?

   a. Tylenol with codeine ¼ grain

   b. Tylenol with codeine ½ grain

   c. Tylenol with codeine 1 grain

Measuring Time and Temperature

UNIT 2

LEARNING OBJECTIVES

1. Convert from military time to the 12-hour clock.
2. Convert from the 12-hour clock to military time.
3. Convert a temperature reading from Fahrenheit to centigrade.
4. Convert a temperature reading from centigrade to Fahrenheit.

Hours, Minutes, and Seconds

Time can be measured using many different units. The basic unit of time is the second. One second is defined as the time needed for a cesium-133 atom to perform 9,192,632,770 complete oscillations, not particularly useful information for most people. A second is about as long as it takes to hiccup. Sixty seconds make a minute, and 60 minutes make an hour. There are 24 hours in a day and 7 days in a week. Although any given month can vary from 28 to 31 days in length, it is common to consider 30 days to count as 1 month. If a pharmacy receives a prescription for a 1-month supply of medication, in most cases the order will be filled with a 30-day supply.

The 24-hour Clock: Military Time

We are accustomed to measuring time in hours after midnight, designated AM and hours after noon, designated PM. For example, 3:00 AM is 3 hours after midnight or 3 o'clock in the morning and 4:00 PM is 4 hours after noon, or 4 o'clock in the afternoon. If the AM or PM designation is left off or if the designation is illegible, there is no way of knowing if the intended time is morning or night. If an evening medication is given in the morning or vice versa, the consequences can endanger the patient. Hospital patients are often on an around the clock dosing schedule, in which the need to distinguish morning and afternoon times is crucial.

To eliminate the need for the AM and PM designation, time is often kept on a 24-hour basis, called **military time**. In military time, all time is measured from midnight, either referred to as 2400 or 0000. Using military time, all times between 0000 and 1159 are between midnight and noon (morning or AM) and all times between 1200 and 2359 are between noon and midnight (afternoon, evening, or PM). Military times are always reported with four digits. To write times from midnight through 9:59 AM, a 0 is used as the first digit. So, 1:30 AM would be reported as 0130 in military time.

Military Time—A time keeping system based on a 24-hour clock.

Rules for conversions using military time

Making the conversion from the usual 12-hour designations to military is fairly easy. Morning times are the same in military time as on the 12-hour clock, except they are written with a zero added to single digit times and the AM designation is eliminated. Just follow these two simple rules for converting PM times.

> **TECH NOTE!**
>
> *To convert a conventional afternoon time (on a 12-hour clock) to military time, add 12 hours.*

> **TECH NOTE!**
>
> *To convert a military time after 1300 to conventional time, subtract 12 hours and add the "PM" designation.*

EXAMPLE

What time is 1730 on a 12-hour clock?

SOLUTION ··

17 is larger than 12, so subtract
1730 − 1200 = 530
Therefore, 1730 is 5:30 PM

EXAMPLE

What time is 0900 (read "oh nine hundred")?

SOLUTION ··

9 is less than 12, so this is a morning time
0900 is 9:00 AM

Measuring Temperatures

Every pharmacy is charged, by a variety of regulatory agencies, with assuring the quality of its medication supplies. As a result, environmental factors like temperature and light exposure must be controlled. Pharmacy technicians are usually asked to monitor and record temperatures in refrigerators, freezers, and medication rooms. In addition, technicians that shelve drug orders must be able to interpret printed temperature ranges so that drugs are properly stored. This means that technicians will need to be familiar with typical temperature ranges for drug storage, and know how to read thermometers.

For example, regulations require medication refrigerators be maintained in a range of 36°F to 46°F. They also require documentation of refrigerator temperatures on a daily basis. When refrigerators are used to store vaccines, the temperatures must be checked twice each day.

NUMBERS AT WORK
Accurate temperature readings of pharmacy equipment such as refrigerators and freezers are essential to maintain drug efficacy and safety.

Fahrenheit and Centigrade

There are several different systems for measuring temperature. Pharmacies may use either **centigrade** or **Fahrenheit**. German physicist, Daniel Fahrenheit, proposed the Fahrenheit temperature scale in 1724. This scale was based on three reference points; 0°F was the temperature of brine, a solution of ice, water, and salt. The temperature of a mixture of ice and water was 32°F and 96°F was the temperature of Mrs. Fahrenheit's armpit. Scientists later slightly redefined the Fahrenheit degree so that the boiling point of water is exactly 180°F higher than its freezing point. On this revised scale, human body temperature is 98.6°F when measured orally (see Table 6-1).

Centigrade—Another name for the celsius temperature scale.

Fahrenheit—A temperature scale in which 32° corresponds to the freezing point of water and 212° corresponds to the boiling point of water.

UNIT **2**

Table 6-1. Temperature Conversions for Common Body Temperatures

Temperatures	Fahrenheit	Centigrade
Oral	98.6°	37°
Rectal or ear	99.7°	37.6°
Axillary (under the arm)	97.6°	36.4°
Fever	100° or more measured orally	37.8° or more

While the above body temperatures are accepted as typical, it is normal for oral, rectal, and axillary temperatures to vary by one degree or more in healthy people.

Andres Celsius (1701–1744), a Swedish astronomer, introduced the centigrade or **Celsius system of temperature measurement**. Celsius based his scale on 100 degrees (hence *centi*-grade) between the freezing point and the boiling point of water at sea level. Interestingly, Celsius designated 0°C as the boiling point and 100°C as the freezing point. In 1744, Swedish botanist Carolus Linneaus reversed this convention by designating the freezing point as 0°C and the boiling point as 100°C. This is the convention we use today. Figure 6-1 shows some common temperatures in the centigrade and Fahrenheit scales.

Celsius System of Temperature Measurement—A temperature scale in which 0° corresponds to the freezing point of water and 100° corresponds to the boiling point of water.

Converting between temperature scales

Because both Fahrenheit and centigrade temperature scales are in common use in the United States, it may be necessary to convert temperatures from centigrade to Fahrenheit or vice versa. If you have access to the Internet or a conversion chart, you can use them for conversions. Otherwise, it is important to be familiar with the calculations used for these conversions.

We use the following formulas for such conversions:

$$C = \frac{F - 32}{1.8} \qquad\qquad F = 1.8\,(C) + 32$$

Figure 6-1. Some common reference temperatures for the centigrade (left) and Fahrenheit (right) scales.

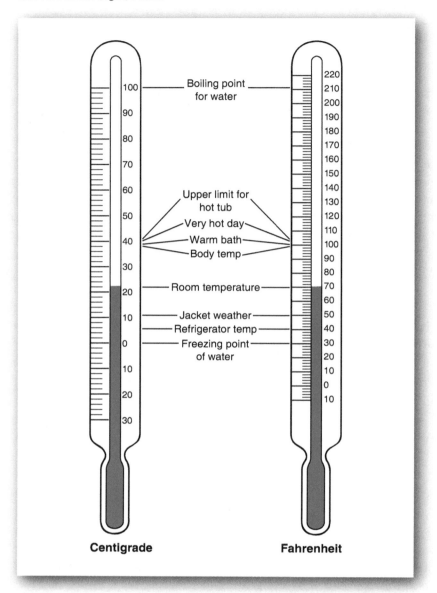

EXAMPLE

Alprostadil injection can be stored for 26 days at 30°C but will last for 34 days if stored at 20°C. At what Fahrenheit temperature must alprostadil injection be stored to last for 34 days?

SOLUTION ·

$F = 1.8\ C + 32$

$F = 1.8(20) + 32$

$F = 36 + 32$

$F = 68$

So alprostadil injection can be stored for 34 days at 68°F, which is cool room temperature.

UNIT 2

EXAMPLE

Ipratropium bromide should be stored at a temperature between 36°F and 77°F. Over what centigrade temperature range should ipratropium bromide be stored?

SOLUTION ··

$$C = \frac{F - 32}{1.8}$$

$$C = \frac{36 - 32}{1.8}$$ $$C = \frac{(77 - 32)}{1.8}$$

$$C = \frac{4}{1.8}$$ $$C = \frac{45}{1.8}$$

$$C = 2.2 \approx 2$$ $$C = 25$$

So, ipratropium bromide should be stored between 2°C and 25°C.

EXAMPLE

A certain laboratory specimen is to be stored at −30°C. What Fahrenheit temperature is this?

SOLUTION ··

$$F = 1.8 (C) + 32$$
$$F = 1.8 (-30) + 32$$
$$F = -22$$

So, the specimen should be stored at −22°F.

Practice Problems

Technician students should use the following problems to get comfortable with typical time and temperature conversions. Understanding these conversions will help you to prepare, deliver, and store medication correctly in the future.

1. Dr. Payne orders penicillin G, 5 million units IVPB to be given to patient Anita Little at 2300 and every 4 hours thereafter throughout the day. At what times on a 12-hour clock should the penicillin IVPB be given?

2. Patient Joe Kerr is in the emergency room for chest pain and reports taking nitroglycerin 0.4 mg sublingually at 9:30 PM and again at 10:00 PM. What times are these in military time?

3. The records indicate that patient Leigh King was admitted to the hospital at 1600. What time is this on a 12-hour clock?

4. Doctor Kauff ordered that a patient be given KCl 20 mEq IVPB at 1300, 1700, and 2100. Nurse Norma Leigh Lucid administered the medication at 1:00 PM, 7:00 PM, and 11:00 PM. Was the medication given at the correct times?

5. Dr. Lance Boyle orders that patient Ann Teac be given furosemide 20 mg PO at 2400 and every 6 hours thereafter for 24 hours. At what military times should the furosemide be given?

6. Normal body temperature, measured orally, is 98.6°F. What is this in degrees centigrade?

7. Normal body temperature, measured rectally, is 37.6°C. What is this in Fahrenheit degrees?

8. Water in an Olympic swimming pool is kept between 25°C and 28°C. What are these temperatures in degrees Fahrenheit?

9. Water droplets in clouds are often super cooled, that is they remain liquid at temperatures below the usual freezing point. A cloud droplet will freeze as soon as its temperature drops below –40°C What is this in degrees Fahrenheit?

10. Plateau Station, Antarctica, recorded a temperature of –86.2°C on July 20, 1968. What is this temperature in degrees Fahrenheit?

11. Sodium bicarbonate should be stored between 15°C and 30°C. What are these temperatures in degrees Fahrenheit?

12. Glucagon should be stored at controlled room temperature between 20°C and 25°C. At what Fahrenheit temperature should glucagon be stored?

13. Diltiazem should be stored at 77°F, but will tolerate temperatures between 59°F and 86°F for brief periods of transport. What are these temperatures in degrees centigrade?

14. Some medications should be stored in a freezer in which the temperature can range from −4°F to 14°F. What are these temperatures in centigrade?

15. Some laboratory specimens must be stored in a freezer in which the temperature ranges from −32°C to −26°C. What are these temperatures in Fahrenheit?

16. Varivax® vaccine should be stored between −15°C and −50°C. The pharmacy freezer reads −10°F. Is it in range?

17. On January 16, 2009, the temperature at Big Black River in Maine was −50°F. What is this temperature in centigrade?

18. In Tipton, Oklahoma, the temperature was 120°F on June 27, 1994. What is this temperature in centigrade?

19. Before it is opened, injectable insulin should be stored at 0°C to 8°C. Should it be stored in the refrigerator, freezer, or at room temperature?

20. To maintain potency, Zostavax® should be stored between −58°F and 5°F. What are these temperatures in degrees centigrade?

Preparing for Problem Solving in Pharmacy

CHAPTER 7

Reading a Prescription

LEARNING OBJECTIVES

1. Identify the required elements of a prescription.
2. Interpret common Latin abbreviations.
3. Transcribe information from a prescription to a prescription label.
4. List three potential sources of error when reading a prescription, creating a label, or selecting a medication.

Introduction

The safety of medication became an issue of public interest in 1937 when a well-respected drug manufacturer developed and marketed a liquid sulfanilamide product dissolved in diethylene glycol (used in antifreeze). Sulfonamides were the first drugs known to treat streptococcal infections in children and adults, and in those days, strep infections were often fatal. Unfortunately, no safety testing was required before drugs were marketed, and prescriptions were not required for purchase of a medication. More than 100 people died, many of them children, from taking this formulation. It was because of this event that the Food and Drug Administration was authorized, and the Federal Food, Drug, and Cosmetic Act written into law. In 1951, the Durham-Humphrey amendment was enacted, which defined two specific categories for medication: prescription drugs and non-prescription, or **over-the-counter (OTC)**, drugs.

What is a prescription?

A **prescription** is a written or electronic order from a physician or other prescriber to the pharmacist, with directions for compounding or dispensing a medication, or providing a device to be used by an individual patient. Typically, prescriptions are written for legend (prescription) medications or devices, but a prescriber can also use them to direct a patient to an OTC product.

> **TECH NOTE!**
>
> **The prescription is a legal record of the communication between prescriber and pharmacist.**

Over-the-Counter Medication— A medication sold without a prescription; for self-use.

While legal requirements of a prescription vary in small ways from state to state, the prescription contains all the information necessary to correctly prepare the medication for a patient's use. Technicians must learn the legal requirements

Prescription—A written or electronic order from a physician or other prescriber to the pharmacist, with directions for preparing a medication or providing a device, to be used by an individual patient.

Strength—Labeled potency of a tablet, capsule, or other drug product.

of this important document in the state where they practice. It is often the responsibility of the technician to provide the initial interpretation of the order so the prescription can be filled and a label produced.

Parts of a Prescription

In order to be safely filled, every prescription must contain certain information. This required information includes the patient's name and address; description of the drug to be dispensed, including name, **strength**, formulation, and quantity; directions to the patient, including the route and frequency of administration; the date (and in an institutional setting, the time) the prescription was written; and the prescriber's signature and other identifying information (see Figure 7-1). When prescriptions are written for use in a hospital setting, they are referred to as *drug orders* and are written differently, but the same essential information is available to the technician and pharmacist through the patient's chart or electronic medical record (see Figure 7-2).

Figure 7-1. A typical prescription format with the essential parts of the prescription shown.

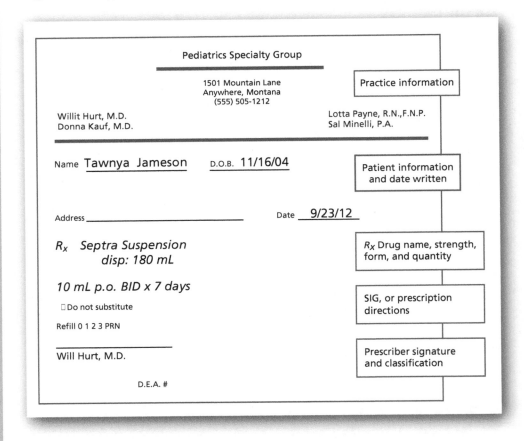

Figure 7-2. Common format of a drug or medication order seen in a hospital.

9/27/12	1. DC warfarin for now	
1315	2. Vitamin K 2.5 mg P.O. x1 now	
	3. Repeat PT/INR in AM	
	4. Protonix 40 mg P.O. q PM	
	Minny Meese, M.D.	
Pt#:059823 RM:9A Rusty Pipes DOB: 2/29/1948 MD: M. Meese		

Prescriber information

Although a legitimate prescription can theoretically be written on any sort of paper, most physicians write prescriptions on prescription pads imprinted with the name, address, and the telephone number of the office, clinic, or hospital where they practice. This information, along with the prescriber's license classification (D.D.S, M.D., D.V.M. or other prescriber type), and the date the prescription was written, is required on a prescription.

The Controlled Substances Act identifies certain drugs for their risk of addiction and potential for abuse. Because of these potential risks, there are additional requirements for prescribing and dispensing medications classified as **controlled substances**. The Drug Enforcement Administration (DEA) assures that these regulations are followed. The prescriber who writes for controlled substances must include his or her DEA registration number on the prescription.

Some states require prescriptions for controlled substances to be written on special, watermarked paper to help prevent forgeries. It is the responsibility of the technician and pharmacist to verify the legitimacy of a prescription for a controlled substance before it is dispensed to the patient, so it is important that you learn any additional requirements imposed by the state where you intend to work.

One important way to verify a prescription's legitimacy is to know the prescriber's handwriting and prescribing practices. Another way is to verify that the DEA number is legitimate. All DEA registration numbers begin with two letters, followed by a seven-digit number. The registration numbers of physicians, dentists, and veterinarians begin with the letters A, B, or F followed by the first letter of the prescriber's last name.

Controlled Substance—A prescription medication identified as having potential for abuse or addiction.

EXAMPLE

A prescribing physician's name is James Doolittle. What could the first letters of a legitimate DEA registration number be?

SOLUTION ···

His DEA number can begin with AD, BD, or FD.

The rest of a DEA number is a series of seven digits. The last digit of these numbers has a relationship to the first six that is always followed (see Table 7-1). If you check the number and it is not correct, then the DEA number is invalid.

EXAMPLE

Dr. Doolittle's DEA number is as follows: BD 2356726. Could this be a legitimate registration number?

SOLUTION ···

1. Add the first, third, and fifth digits
   $$2 + 5 + 7 = 14$$
2. Add the second, fourth, and sixth digits
   $$3 + 6 + 2 = 11$$
3. Multiply the sum determined in Step 2 by 2
   $$11 \times 2 = 22$$
4. Add the total from Steps 1 and 3
   $$22 + 14 = 36$$
5. Verify that the last digit of the sum of Steps 1 and 3 (6) is the same as the last digit in the registration number, BD 2356726. Since the verification number checks out, this could be a legitimate DEA number.

Table 7-1. Method That Verifies a DEA Number Is Not Invalid

1. Add the first, third, and fifth numbers of the seven-digit DEA registration number.
2. Now add the second, fourth, and sixth numbers.
3. Double the sum you just calculated in Step 2.
4. Add the total from Step 1 and Step 3. The last digit in the sum of Steps 1 and 3 must match the seventh digit in the DEA number; it is called the "checksum" number.

NUMBERS AT WORK

Accurate math is important in the identification and verification of DEA numbers and legitimate prescriptions.

Patient information

Every prescription must include enough information to identify the patient for whom it is intended. In most states this includes first and last name, and address. States usually allow pharmacy personnel to fill in a patient's address. Some states may require additional information, such as the age of the patient. Most community and all hospital pharmacies supplement required data with a patient profile that includes information crucial to the safe dispensing of medication, such as the patient's height, weight, age, sex, and allergies.

Hospital order forms are labeled with patient name and identification number, along with date of birth, the admitting physician's name, or other institution-specific information. Pharmacy employees access the patient's electronic record for the purpose of entering or preparing drug orders by using the patient identification number or other form of hospital ID.

R_X: Drug name, strength, formulation, and quantity

The main body of the prescription, traditionally referred to as the inscription and subscription, includes the name, strength, and the desired formulation of the drug (such as tablet or capsule), and any directions to the pharmacist for compounding purposes. This information is often preceded by the symbol R_X, an abbreviation for the Latin "*recipe.*" The symbol R_X was traditionally interpreted to mean, "take thou," the direction to the pharmacist to produce the prescription for the patient, usually by mixing, or compounding, the ingredients according to the art and science of pharmacy practice. To **compound** means to prepare a product from pharmaceutical ingredients.

In modern community pharmacy practice, it is unusual for pharmacists or technicians to compound medications on a regular basis. However, there are compounding pharmacies that prepare specialty non-sterile products for outpatient use in a growing number of communities. Table 7-2 lists some of the Latin abbreviations that may be used in directions for compounded products. Sterile compounding of products for intravenous administration is routinely done in hospitals and in home-health pharmacies.

Compound—To prepare a product from pharmaceutical ingredients.

Table 7-2. Common Abbreviations Used in Compounding and Their Meanings

Abbreviation	Latin/Early Meaning	Common Usage
aa	ana	Of each
ad	ad	Up to
aq	aqua	Aqueous, water
disp.		Dispense
comp.		Compound
d.t.d.	dentur tales doses	Dispense such doses
mist.	mistura	Mix
non rep.	non repetatur	Do not repeat; no refills
pulv.	pulvis, pulveris	Powder
q.s.	quantum sufficiat	A sufficient quantity
sol.	solutio	Solution
ss	semis	One half
ung	unguentum	Ointment
u.d. or ut. dict.	ut dictum	As directed

Sig: Directions for use

The **signa or sig** is the area of the prescription that provides directions to the patient on how to use the medication, and is decoded and transcribed onto the prescription label. This information indicates how much of the medication the patient is to take, for example one tablet or two. The directions include the route of administration, such as by mouth, apply to the skin, or other ways of administering a medication. Frequency of administration is another important part of these instructions. In some cases, directions may include other special instructions, such as removing a topical medication after a certain time period.

The sig is nearly always written using common Latin prescription abbreviations. As the technician, you must be absolutely certain of the directions before you enter the information into a computer system or type a label. If you are unsure of the meaning of abbreviations or have any other concerns about the dose or directions, ask before you proceed to fill the prescription.

> ## ▶ TECH NOTE!
>
> *"When in doubt, check it out" is the rule to follow before you fill any prescription or drug order.*

Interpreting and Transcribing Prescriptions

Common Latin and other medical abbreviations

Latin abbreviations were originally used in pharmacy as a short cut to writing out lengthy directions to the pharmacist, and also to assure that patients remained unaware of their conditions and treatments. Now that health care providers and patients agree that it is both the right and responsibility of patients to be as informed as possible about their health, these abbreviations are used as a prescription shorthand and out of habit.

There is not really any way to avoid memorizing these abbreviations. If you speak Spanish or Italian, or took Latin at some point in your education, they may make more sense and be easier to remember, although some abbreviations used in health care are not Latin based. Table 7-3 lists some of the most common abbreviations used in prescription or drug order writing.

Calculating prescription quantities

Sometimes, rather than indicate a number of tablets or capsules to dispense, a prescriber will write the quantity to be dispensed as number of days supply. The pharmacy personnel must then determine the quantity of medication to prepare. This way of writing a prescription can make it difficult to determine the necessary quantity for medications prescribed "as needed," but is otherwise a straightforward calculation. First, determine the number of doses the patient is to take in 1 day. Then multiply the number of doses/day times the number of days to be supplied.

Table 7-3. Frequently Used Prescription Abbreviations and Medical Terminology

Abbreviation	Latin	Meaning	Abbreviation	Latin	Meaning
			**Dosage Forms and Routes of Administration**		
cap		capsule	a.d	auris dextro	right ear
gtt(s)	gutta(e)	drop(s)	a.s.	auris sinistro	left ear
liq	liquor	Solution or liquid	a.u.	auris utro	both ears
lot.		lotion	bucc	buccal	in the cheek
supp.		suppository	IM		intramuscular
syr.		syrup	inj		injection
sol.		solution	IV		intravenous
susp.		suspension	IVP		IV push
tab		tablet	IVPB		IV piggyback
tr, tinc.		tincture	o.d.	oculo dextro	right eye
			o.s.	oculo sinistro	left eye
			o.u.	oculo utro	both eyes
			p.o.	per os	by mouth
			p.r.		per rectum
			sc or sq		subcutaneous
			Top.		topical
		Frequency			
a.c.	ante cibum	before meals	p.m.	postmeridian	afternoon
ad. lib.	ad libitum	as desired	p.r.n.	pro re nata	as needed
a.m.	antemeridian	morning	q	quaque	every
B.I.D.	bis in die	twice a day	q.d.	quaque die	daily
H.S.		at bedtime	q.i.d.	quater in die	four times a day
h		hour	q4h		every 4 hours*
min.		minute	q.o.d.		every other day
noct.	nocte	night	stat		immediately
p.c.	post cibum	after meals	t.i.d	ter in die	three times a day
		Other Common Abbreviations			
a	ante	before	NKA		no known allergies
asap		as soon as possible	NPO		nothing by mouth
BM		bowel movement	NS		normal saline
BP		blood pressure	n/v		nausea/vomiting
DC or d/c		discontinue	p	post	after
dx		diagnosis	S.O.B.		shortness of breath
HA		headache	URI		upper respiratory infection
L or R		left or right	UTI		urinary tract infection
M.R.		may repeat			

*Any number can be used here, e.g., q12h means every 12 hours.

> **EXAMPLE**
>
> You receive a prescription for Septra DS® as follows:
>
> *Rx:* Septra DS tabs
>
> 10-day supply
>
> *Sig:* i tablet BID
>
> How many tablets will you dispense?
>
> **SOLUTION** •
>
> First, determine the number of doses per day. BID means twice a day, so the patient will receive two doses, of one tablet apiece, each day. Next, calculate the total tablets for 10 days.
>
> 2 tabs/day × 10 days = 20 tablets
>
> Now look at an example where the total number of doses per day is not quite so obvious.

> **EXAMPLE**
>
> A physician orders Robitussin AC® cough syrup for 15-year-old Dunmore Coffin, who is to take 5 mL every 4 hours if needed for cough. The prescription directs you to dispense a 5-day supply. The pharmacist asks that you assume Dunmore will take the medication around the clock. How much Robitussin AC® will you dispense?
>
> **SOLUTION** •
>
> There are 24 hours per day and the medication may be taken every 4 hours.
>
> Doses/day = 24 hours/day × 1 dose/4 hours = 6 doses/day
>
> Solution needed = 5 mL/dose × 6 doses/day × 5 days = 150 mL

Preparing a label from a prescription

Correct labeling of a prescription is important for many reasons. It is the link that connects the prescriber's order, the pharmacy's product, and the patient's use of the treatment at home. When preparing a prescription for outpatient use, the label must bear the prescription number that is assigned when the prescription is filled. Other required label information includes the date filled, the drug name, strength, and quantity, the initials of the person who filled it, and an expiration date for the medication. Most importantly, the label includes directions to the patient on the correct use of the drug. Prescription label requirements are determined by individual states, but a typical label is represented in Figure 7-3.

Pharmacy personnel must decode the Latin abbreviations on the written prescription into simple, unambiguous language for the label. It is essential that the prescription label be written in language that anyone can understand, since pharmacy staff usually does not know the education level of the patient for whom the prescription is intended. In some situations, the prescription label may need to be translated into another language. Assuring that patients understand the prescription label is the first step toward correct medication use.

Figure 7-3. Format of a typical outpatient prescription label.

Bellis' Santa Maria Drug Store
522 N. Broadway, Santa Maria, CA
(805) 555-1212

Rx 123456   Dr. Brown

Ron A. Way   1/15/12 RPH

48 Methotrexate 2.5 mg Tablets (BB)

Take four tablets by mouth every Monday for rheumatoid arthritis.

No refills   Exp: 10/29/13

Yellow, scored oval tablet imprinted with B572

In hospitals, a nurse most often administers the medication to the patient, so labeling requirements are different than for home use. Medications purchased from the manufacturer in **unit-dose** packaging (single-dose packages) are already labeled, but compounded IV solutions and multi-dose oral, topical, or inhaled products are labeled in the pharmacy. Hospital labeling includes additional information, such as patient room number, dosing schedule, and for IV solutions, infusion rates.

Although the Latin sig on a prescription contains no verb, action can be inferred from the route of administration. For an oral medication, the directions on a prescription label will begin with the verb "take." Directions for a topical medication might begin with "apply." In addition, the dose must be written in the most understandable terms possible. For example, a dose of 15 mL should be written as "1 tablespoonful" followed by 15 mL in parentheses. Look over the following examples to make sure you understand this concept.

> **Unit-Dose System**—A system of drug dispensing where a 24-hour supply of medication is dispensed in ready-to-use, single-use dose packages.

EXAMPLE 1

Decode the following prescription language and write the instructions in simple English.

Rx: Digoxin solution 0.05 mg/1 mL

Sig: 0.25 mg p.o. QAM

SOLUTION ···

Because the product is taken P.O. (by mouth) we will use the verb "take" in transcribing these directions. You will also need to change the dose from 0.25 mg to a measurement more easily understood by the patient. You will need to determine how many mL will contain the dose 0.25 mg.

$$\frac{0.05 \text{ mg}}{1 \text{ mL}} \times (\text{desired vol}) = 0.25 \text{ mg}$$

Desired volume = 5 mL

So the patient directions should read:

Take 1 teaspoonful (5 mL) by mouth every morning.

EXAMPLE 2

Decode the following and write the instructions in simple English.

Rx: Gentamicin Ophth.

Sig: gtts ii o.s. q6h x 5 days

SOLUTION ···

For an eye or ear medication use the verbs "instill," "use," or "place" for the directions, and specify the site of administration.

Instill two drops in the left eye every 6 hours for 5 days. OR

Use two drops in the left eye every 6 hours for 5 days. OR

Place two drops in the left eye every 6 hours for 5 days.

EXAMPLE 3

Decode the following sig and write directions in simple English.

Rx: Lantus insulin 100 units/mL 1 vial

Sig: 10 units s.c. QHS

SOLUTION ···

For an injectable medication use the verbs "inject" or "give" in the directions and indicate how or where to give the medication.

Inject 10 units under the skin of the abdomen or thigh every night at bedtime.

or

Give 10 units under the skin of the abdomen or thigh every night at bedtime.

NUMBERS AT WORK

Understanding the relationships between medication forms, dosing amounts, and dosing instructions is key to accurate dosing.

Medication Errors in the Pharmacy

Potential sources of error when interpreting prescriptions

Many commercially available prescription drugs are sold in a variety of formulations and strengths, which creates potential for confusion. For example a product might be available as tablets in a number of strengths, liquid, and **delayed-release** tablets (a formulation designed to release medication slowly). As the technician, you need to know which formulation is the right one. A delayed-release product cannot be substituted for a product that dissolves immediately, even if the strength is the same, and the reverse is also true.

Delayed-Release—A dosage form that releases medication at a later time or over an extended period of time.

EXAMPLE

If the following drug order was written in a hospital, could you fill it without some clarification from the pharmacist, physician, or nurse?

6/15/12	Furosemide 20 mg by mouth this AM	
0915	and tomorrow AM for edema.	
	James B. Little, MD	
Pt#: 243786 RM:4A Jonathan Jump MD: Little DOB: 2/29/2005		

SOLUTION ···

Furosemide is available in two different oral formulations that would be appropriate for a child Jonathan's age (note: DOB means date of birth). If he can swallow small tablets, then a tablet is appropriate. If not, furosemide is available in a liquid formulation. Clarification is necessary.

Illegible prescriber handwriting is another source of errors in pharmacy. Some prescribers are notorious for their bad handwriting. To prevent interpretation errors, many physicians, hospitals and clinics are now moving to electronic prescription writing and computerized prescriber order entry.

▶ **TECH NOTE!**

If any part of a prescription is unclear, it is the responsibility of the technician to ask for clarification by the pharmacist before filling it.

Error-prone abbreviations

Some abbreviations are considered risky to use because they are easily misinterpreted. For example the abbreviations QD (daily) can be interpreted as QID (four times daily), or QOD (every other day) especially if the prescriber's handwriting is bad. The Joint Commission, which determines whether hospitals are accredited, designates these confusing abbreviations as unapproved and has placed them on an official "Do Not Use" list (available at www.jointcommission.org/assets/1/18/dnu_list.pdf). Although these unapproved abbreviations are deemed unsafe in hospitals, they still are used for prescriptions where oversight agencies have no jurisdiction (retail pharmacies), and you will need to know how to read them. Unapproved abbreviations are listed in Table 7-4.

Table 7-4. Official "Do Not Use" Abbreviations with Potential Problems and Correct Alternatives

"Do Not Use" Abbreviations

Do Not Use	Potential Problem	Use Instead
U	Mistaken for "0," the number 4, or cc	Unit or units
I.U.	Mistaken for IV or the number 10	International units
QD, Q.D. QOD, Q.O.D.	Mistaken for each other or Q.I.D.	Daily Every other day
Trailing zero (X.0 mg) Lack of leading zero (.Xmg)	Decimal point is missed, possible ten-fold dosing error	X mg 0.X mg
MS	Can mean morphine sulfate or magnesium sulfate	Morphine sulfate
MSO4, MgSO4	Confused with one another	Magnesium sulfate or morphine sulfate

Possible Future "Do Not Use" Additions

Do Not Use	Potential Problem	Use Instead
> (greater than) < (less than)	Misinterpreted as number 7 or letter L, confused with one another	Greater than, less than
Abbreviations for drug names	Misinterpreted because there are similar abbreviations for multiple drugs	Write out the drug name in full
Apothecary units such as grain, dram	Confused with metric units	Metric units
cc	Mistaken for U, 00	mL, ml, or milliliters
μg	Mistaken for mg, resulting in 1,000-fold overdose	mcg or micrograms

Source: From the Joint Commission Official List.

Look-alike, sound-alike drug names and packaging

The drug name and manufacturer packaging are another possible source of confusion. Some drugs have names that look similar to other drug names, especially if the handwriting on the prescription is unclear. The manufacturer's label on one drug package can look just like another package of a different strength. Drugs with these confusing names and labels are referred to as look-alike, sound-alike drugs. When taking a medication off the shelf, the technicians must always read the label in order to assure that the correct drug, formulation, and strength was selected.

▶ *TECH NOTE!*

When selecting a medication, read the label!

Look-alike, sound-alike errors can be extremely serious, as in the case of well-known actor Dennis Quaid's newborn twins, who nearly died when they received a 1000-fold overdose of the anticoagulant heparin. A pharmacy technician placed vials of heparin 10,000 units/mL into the automated dispensing cabinet where the 10 units/mL heparin should have been. The similar size and labeling of the vial was part of the reason this error was made. In addition, the nurse that gave the drug did not read the label.

These are just some of the possible ways that errors can be made when dispensing medications. A good work ethic, an understanding of the problem of medication errors, and knowledge of the medications and processes in the pharmacy where you work will be your best defense against making errors. It is important to remember that every employee in a pharmacy shares in the responsibility of getting the correct drug to every patient.

▶ **TECH NOTE!**

Every employee in a pharmacy shares in the responsibility of getting the correct drug to the patient.

Practice Problems

1. List eight pieces of information required on a prescription.

2. Write the meaning of the following abbreviations used in compounding:
   a. qs   b. ad   c. aa   d. comp.

3. Write the meaning of the following routes of administration:
   a. p.o.   b. IVP   c. IM   d. top

4. Decode the following prescription directions and write a simple sentence in English as it would appear on the label.
   a. i tab p.o. b.i.d.
   b. ii caps p.o. q6h ×7 days
   c. Lantus Insulin 100 units/mL
      sig: 20 units s.c. qAM
   d. Cortisporin Otic® gtts disp: 15 mL
      sig: gtts iii a.s. t.i.d. 5 days. Place cotton in L canal $\bar{p}$ gtts.

5. Interpret the following drug orders as a nurse might read them and write out your interpretation.
   a. Zosyn 2.25 g IVPB Q8H
   b. Morphine sulfate 5 mg sc q3H prn moderate pain or S.O.B.
   c. NS 1000 mL IV to run at 125 mL/hr
   d. Naloxone 0.4 mg IVP stat and q 15–30 min prn respiratory depression

6. Why is each of the following abbreviations on the "Do Not Use" list? Explain the potential problem for each dangerous abbreviation and the safe alternative.
   a. QD
   b. trailing zero (i.e., 4.0 mg)
   c. U
   d. lack of a leading zero (i.e., .4 mg)

7. Check the following DEA numbers to see if they meet the test for validity. Indicate why you think they could be valid or are invalid.
   a. Wilma Ruth, M.D., DEA Registration # A.R. 1234563
   b. Daniel Bones, M.D., DEA Registration # B.D. 2754388
   c. Rebecca Darling, D.V.M., DEA Registration # B.D 5704386

8. A prescription for Tylenol® with codeine liquid for Jonathan Jameson, who broke his leg when he fell off the monkey bars, instructs the parents to give their child 5 mL every 4 hours if needed for pain. The physician wants the pharmacy to dispense a 5-day supply. How much should the pharmacy dispense? Assume the child takes the medication as ordered, around the clock.

9. Write the abbreviations that correspond to the following words or phrases.
   a. capsule
   b. suspension
   c. after meals

    d. twice a day

    e. as directed

    f. no known allergies

10. Lantus® Insulin contains 100 units per mL and is sold in a 10-mL vial. If a patient injects 15 units (0.15 mL) QHS at what time of day will he be administering the insulin? How much insulin will he use in 1 week?

11. Lantus® Insulin expires 28 days after the vial is opened. If the patient in Problem 10 uses his insulin as ordered, how much will be left in the vial after 28 days?

12. What information is needed before you can fill the following prescription?

Dan Kashain, M.D.
1689 South Court Street, Visalia, CA

Name: Carter Moss

Address: 15510 Ave 313, Visalia, CA

Date: 2/29/12

Rx: Azithromycin 250 mg/5 mL

Sig: i tsp q 6

Refills: -0-

Dan Kashain   M.D.

---

13. List four routes of administration by which medication may be administered.

14. List three causes of errors that can occur while filling a prescription and three corresponding methods for preventing the error.

15. Write out the directions listed below completely, as you would type them on a prescription label.

    a. ii gtts o.s. qid while awake

    b. 15 mL p.o. q4h prn cough or congestion

    c. i tab sl q 5 min × 3 prn chest pain

    d. caps ii PO B.I.D for blood pressure

16. Write the meaning of the following abbreviations.

    a. oz

    b. AC and HS

    c. q8h

    d. prn

    e. au

    f. qs

17. Calculate the number of tablets needed to fill the following prescription.

Rx: Azithromycin 250 mg tablets

Disp: 5 day supply

Sig: tabs ii now, then i tab daily

18. For the following drug order:
    Vancomycin 1 g IVPB Q 12H × 6 weeks for osteomyelitis
    a. How many IVPB doses will the patient receive daily?
    b. How many doses will the patient receive over the entire course of therapy?

19. You receive the following prescription for amoxicillin suspension for a child with an acute middle ear infection:
    Amoxicillin susp. 400 mg/5 mL
    320 mg (4 mL) Q8H ×7 days
    Amoxicillin 400 mg/5 mL for suspension is available in 50 mL, 75 mL, and 100 mL bottles. Which size will you dispense?

20. The automated dispensing cabinet in the ICU needs to be filled with enough hydromorphone 1-mg vials to last the next 24 hours. Three patients in the unit have the following orders:

    Patient A: Hydromorphone 1 mg Q4H prn moderate pain
    Patient B: Hydromorphone 1 mg Q2H prn moderate to severe pain
    Patient C: Hydromorphone 0.5 mg Q3H for pain
    Assume that each patient will take the maximum dose allowed. There are 12 vials available in the unit at present. Partial vials cannot be saved for another dose.
    a. How many total vials are needed for 24 hours?
    b. How many more hydromorphone vials will you need to add to last 24 hours?

21. For each of the sigs given below, state how many doses the patient will receive in 1 day.
    a. Q2h
    b. TID
    c. Q8h

22. What is the maximum number of doses/day the patient should take for these sigs?
    a. Q4H prn
    b. Q3H prn, max 6 doses/day
    c. Q2H while awake (assume patient sleeps 8 hours)

23. The pharmacist receives the following prescription for compounding:

Drug A	60 mL
Drug B	500 mg
Alcohol 70%	60 mL
Lotion C qs ad	200 mL

    a. What does qs ad mean?
    b. The pharmacy has a 6-ounce bottle of lotion C on the shelf. Will that be enough to compound the prescription?

24. How many tablets or capsules will be dispensed with each of the following prescriptions?
    a. Tetracycline 250-mg capsules
       one BID for acne
       disp: 1 month's supply

   b. Lomotil tabs
      q3h prn diarrhea, max 6/day
      disp: 1 week supply
   c. Ampicillin 500-mg capsules, take 2 grams 30 minutes before dental
      procedures on Monday and Thursday this week, and Tuesday next week.

25. **For each of the past 4 weeks, the usage of Vicodin® tablets from the automated dispensing cabinet you fill is as follows:**

Week 1: 86 tablets   **Week 3: 93 tablets**
Week 2: 120 tablets   **Week 4: 112 tablets**

   a. How many Vicodin® tablets are used in an average week?
   b. The current tablet count in the drawer is 7 tablets and the maximum for
      the drawer is 125 tablets. How many tablets should you add to reach the
      maximum?

CHAPTER 8

Using Critical Thinking to Solve Problems

LEARNING OBJECTIVES

1. Define *equation*.
2. Solve an equation using addition or subtraction.
3. Solve an equation using multiplication or division.
4. Identify the variable in a word problem.
5. Translate a word problem into an equation.
6. Estimate an answer, and check for reasonableness when solving a word problem.

UNIT 3

Introduction

Now that you can read a prescription and do conversions from one system of weights and measures to another, you are ready to apply these mathematical skills to solving problems in real pharmacy settings. You will learn to estimate solutions to such problems before proceeding with a mathematical solution. Then you will learn to translate a word problem or situation into a mathematical equation, solve the equation and check the solution against that initial estimate for reasonableness. This check for reasonableness is an essential step in catching mathematical errors that can translate to drug errors. Catching these errors before they reach a patient can mean the difference between life and death.

Equations and Unknowns

An **equation** is a mathematical statement of equality. Every equation contains an equal sign. Many equations state a numerical fact.

Example: $1 + 2 = 3$ $5 - 1 = 4$
$3 \times 4 = 12$ $21 \div 3 = 7$

Sometimes an equation will contain an unknown, or a variable. A **variable** is a symbol for a number we don't yet know. Any letter or symbol can be chosen as the variable. Very often, the letter "x" is chosen, but it may be helpful to choose a letter that reminds you of the units you are seeking. For example, you could use N to represent the number of tablets. The purpose of solving the equation is to determine the value of the variable. The correct value for the variable makes the equation a true mathematical statement.

Equation—A mathematical statement of equality.

Variable—The letter or symbol used to represent an unknown quantity.

Solving equations using addition, subtraction, multiplication, or division

The goal in solving an equation is to determine the value of the variable. To accomplish that, isolate the variable, that is, separate the variable so that it is alone on one side of the equal sign, with a number on the other side. If the variable is not alone, because, for example, another number is added to the variable, we subtract that number from each side of the equal sign.

> **TECH NOTE!**
>
> *When solving equations, any operation you perform on one side of the equation must be performed on the other side of the equation.*

EXAMPLE

$x + 5 = 7$

SOLUTION ···

$x + 5 = 7$
$x + 5 - 5 = 7 - 5$
$x = 2$
We can check our solution by substituting this value for the variable in the original equation, then checking that both sides of the equal sign are the same.
$2 + 5 = 7$
$7 = 7$

EXAMPLE

$x + 9 = 21$

SOLUTION ···

$x + 9 = 21$
$x + 9 - 9 = 21 - 9$
$x = 12$
Check
$12 + 9 = 21$
$21 = 21$

If the variable is not alone due to a number that is subtracted, we add that number to each side of the equal sign.

EXAMPLE

$x - 7 = 13$

SOLUTION ···

$x - 7 = 13$
$x - 7 + 7 = 13 + 7$
$x = 20$

Check
20 – 7 = 13
13 = 13

Sometimes the variable in an equation is multiplied by a number. To indicate that a variable is multiplied by a number, we write the number to the left of the variable.

EXAMPLE

$3x$ means three times x

SOLUTION ·

$\frac{2}{3}x$ means two thirds times x or two thirds of x

If a variable is multiplied by a number, we can isolate the variable by dividing by that number on both sides of the equal sign. When solving such an equation, we use the fraction bar to indicate division.

EXAMPLE

$3x = 21$

SOLUTION ·

Solve   Check
$3x = 21$ $3 \times 7 = 21$
$\dfrac{3x}{3} = \dfrac{21}{3}$ $21 = 21$
$x = 7$

If our unknown is multiplied by a fraction, we must multiply by the fraction's reciprocal on each side to solve the equation. To find the reciprocal, invert (exchange the numerator and denominator) the fraction.

EXAMPLE

$\frac{2}{3}x = 16$

SOLUTION ·

$\frac{2}{3}x = 16$

$\frac{3}{2} \times \frac{2}{3}x = \frac{3}{2} \times 16$

$x = 24$

Remember that the reciprocal of 0.1 or $\frac{1}{10}$ is 10, the reciprocal of 0.01 or $\frac{1}{100}$ is 100 and the reciprocal of 0.001 or $\frac{1}{1000}$ is 1000.

EXAMPLE

$0.01x = 23$

SOLUTION $\cdots\cdots\cdots\cdots\cdots\cdots\cdots\cdots\cdots\cdots\cdots\cdots\cdots\cdots\cdots\cdots\cdots\cdots\cdots\cdots$

$0.01x = 23$
$100 \times 0.01x = 100 \times 23$
$x = 2300$

When a variable is multiplied by a number and has a number added or subtracted, eliminate the added or subtracted number first, then the number that is multiplied.

EXAMPLE

$3x + 5 = 11$

SOLUTION $\cdots\cdots\cdots\cdots\cdots\cdots\cdots\cdots\cdots\cdots\cdots\cdots\cdots\cdots\cdots\cdots\cdots\cdots\cdots\cdots$

$3x + 5 = 11$
$3x + 5 - 5 = 11 - 5$
$3x = 6$
$\dfrac{3x}{3} = \dfrac{6}{3}$
$x = 2$

To check your solution, substitute the answer you get for the variable in the original equation and simplify.

$3(2) + 5 = 11$
$6 + 5 = 11$
$11 = 11$

EXAMPLE

$\dfrac{2}{3}x - 7 = 15$

SOLUTION $\cdots\cdots\cdots\cdots\cdots\cdots\cdots\cdots\cdots\cdots\cdots\cdots\cdots\cdots\cdots\cdots\cdots\cdots\cdots\cdots$

$\dfrac{2}{3}x - 7 = 15$

$\dfrac{2}{3}x - 7 + 7 = 15 + 7$

$\dfrac{2}{3}x = 22$

$\dfrac{3}{2} \times \dfrac{2}{3}x = \dfrac{3}{2} \times 22$

$x = 33$

Check

$\frac{2}{3}(33) - 7 = 15$

$22 - 7 = 15$

$15 = 15$

EXAMPLE

$0.1x + 5 = 35$

SOLUTION

$0.1x + 5 = 35$

$0.1x + 5 - 5 = 35 - 5$

$0.1x = 30$

$10 \times 0.1x = 10 \times 30$

$x = 300$

Check

$0.1 \times 300 + 5 = 35$

$30 + 5 = 35$

$35 = 35$

Word Problems

As a pharmacy technician, you will seldom be handed a mathematical equation to solve. Rather, there will be situations that require you to find an unknown quantity. This unknown quantity can be represented by a variable. First, translate the situation into an equation. Then, you can solve the equation and check to see if your answer makes sense in the context of the situation.

The first step of this process, defining the variable, is extremely important, so we will devote some time to practicing that step. In the following situations, define the variable (identify the unknown quantity).

EXAMPLE

Define the variable:

The doctor prescribes 500 mg of ciprofloxacin to be given every 12 hours. The pharmacy only stocks 250-mg tablets. How many 250-mg tablets of ciprofloxacin should be given at each administration?

SOLUTION

Let n (our variable) = the number of 250-mg ciprofloxacin tablets to be given at each administration.

EXAMPLE

Define the variable:

Two tablets of 250 mg ciprofloxacin are given as one dose. How many milligrams of ciprofloxacin are given per dose?

SOLUTION ···

Let m = milligrams of ciprofloxacin in each dose.

EXAMPLE

Define the variable:

Two 250-mg ciprofloxacin tablets are to be given every 12 hours. How many ciprofloxacin tablets are given in a day?

SOLUTION ···

Let n = the number of ciprofloxacin tablets given in a day.

Notice that the variable must always represent something that is quantified as a number. Each of the three situations involves ciprofloxacin, but the variable was never just "ciprofloxacin." The variable also included units, either tablets or milligrams.

Once the unknown is identified, it is important to make an estimate of the answer. An estimate is based upon common sense and the information that you are given in the problem or situation. The easiest way to estimate is to round the numbers in the problem. If you are working with decimals, round to the nearest whole number. If you are working with larger quantities (i.e., 38) round to the nearest multiple of five or ten. In the following situations, define the variable (identify the unknown quantity). Then make an estimate of the answer.

EXAMPLE

A pharmacy stocks 910 tablets of a certain medication. Two thirds of these tablets are used to fill prescriptions. How many tablets remain?

SOLUTION ···

Identify the unknown. Let x = the number of tablets that remain.

Next, estimate the answer. Round 910 to 900. If 2/3 of the tablets are used, then 1/3 remains, and 1/3 of 900 is 300. Since we rounded down, we have underestimated the answer by a small amount. The number of tablets that remain should be a little more than 300.

Once the variable is appropriately defined, we must translate English words and phrases into mathematical expressions. Table 8-1 shows a partial list of verbal phrases used to indicate different mathematical operations. The words "is" or "are" in a problem are represented by an equal sign.

Table 8-1. Translating Word Problems Into Equations

Math Operation	Related Words	When a Problem Says . . .	The Mathematical Expression Is . . .
Addition	the sum of	the sum of 7 and a number	$X + 7$
	increased by	a number increased by 5	$X + 5$
	the total	the total of 4 and a number	$4 + X$
	more than	6 more than a number	$6 + X$
Subtraction	the difference between	the difference between X and 2	$X - 2$
		the difference between 7 and X	$7 - X$
	less than	5 less than a number	$X - 5$
	decreased by	a number decreased by 8	$X - 8$
Multiplication	times	9 times a number	$9X$
	the product of	the product of 7 and a number	$7X$
		two thirds of a number	$\frac{2}{3}X$
	twice	twice a number	$2X$
	double	double a quantity	$2X$
Division	divided by	A number divided by 3	$\frac{X}{3}$
	quotient of	5 divided by a number	$\frac{5}{X}$
	the ratio of	the quotient of 7 and a number	$\frac{7}{X}$
		the quotient of a number and 8	$\frac{X}{8}$
		the ratio of 9 to a number	$\frac{9}{X}$
		the ratio of a number to 6	$\frac{X}{6}$

> ► **TECH NOTE!**
>
> **The word "is" translates to an equal sign.**

Notice that there are mathematical operations in which the order we solve does matter and those in which order does not matter. Addition and multiplication are commutative (can be completed in any order), but subtraction and division are not.

Translate the following situations into an algebraic equation with a variable.

EXAMPLE

A pharmacy has 6 ounces of Hycodan® on the shelf. Sixteen more ounces of Hycodan® are delivered to the pharmacy. What is the total number of ounces of Hycodan® in the pharmacy after the delivery?

SOLUTION ·

Let x = the total number of ounces of Hycodan® after the delivery.
6 oz + 16 oz = x

EXAMPLE

After 30 diazepam 5-mg tablets are used to fill a prescription, the pharmacy has 360 tablets left. What was the original number of diazepam 5-mg tablets?

SOLUTION ·

Let x = the original number of diazepam 5-mg tablets.
$x - 30 = 360$

Now, let's look at some pharmacy situations, estimate a solution, translate the situation into an equation, solve the equation, and check our solution against the initial estimate for reasonableness.

EXAMPLE

A pharmacy has 940 levothyroxine 100-mcg tablets on the shelf. The pharmacy receives three orders for 30 levothyroxine 100-mcg tablets.

A. After filling these prescriptions, how many levothyroxine tablets remain on the pharmacy shelf?

B. How many prescriptions of 30 tablets can be filled with the remaining supply of levothyroxine 100-mcg tablets?

SOLUTION ·

Estimate first. We can round 940 to 950. 950 minus 90 tablets for the prescriptions leaves 860. Since we rounded up, this is an overestimate, and our answer should be a little less than 860.

A. Define the variable: Let x = the number of levothyroxine tablets remaining on the shelf.
Translate to an equation:
$940 - 3(30) = x$
Solve equation:
$940 - 90 = x$
$850 = x$

B. These 850 tablets are to be *divided* into prescriptions of 30 tablets each.
$$\frac{850}{30} = 28.33$$
So 28 more prescriptions of 30 levothyroxine 100-mcg tablets can be filled.

Practice Problems

Solve the following equations:

1. $\dfrac{1}{10}x = 25$

2. $0.001x = 325$

3. $100x = 50$

4. $x - 5 = 235$

5. $30x + 15 = 345$

Identify the unknown (define the variable) in the following situations.

6. A prescription requires that amoxicillin 500 mg be given three times daily for 10 days. Amoxicillin is available in 500-mg capsules. How many capsules are needed to fill the prescription?

7. Ritalin® is available in 20-mg scored tablets. How many tablets should be given per dose if the dose is 30 mg?

8. A prescription calls for 5 mg of Valium® to be taken twice daily. How many grams of Valium® will the patient take in 30 days?

9. A prescription calls for 40 mg of furosemide to be given four times daily. How many milligrams of furosemide will be taken daily?

10. A prescription calls for 10 mg of Inderal® to be taken three times daily. How many milligrams of Inderal® will the patient take in 30 days?

Identify the unknown (define the variable) in the following situations. Make an estimate of the answer.

11. A prescription for risperidone 1 mg calls for one tablet three times daily for one day, then two tablets twice a day for 1 day, then three tablets twice a day for 7 days. How many tablets are needed to fill the prescription?

12. Tetracycline is available in 250-mg capsules. A prescription calls for two capsules four times a day for 10 days, then one capsule four times a day for 20 days. How many milligrams of tetracycline will the patient ingest over 30 days?

13. A prescription calls for one tablet to be taken four times a day. Ninety tablets are dispensed. How many days should this prescription last?

14. A pharmacy stocks 124 bottles of vitamins on the shelf. One third of these are destroyed because they are past the "use by" date. How many bottles are destroyed?

15. Seventy-two percent of a 500 mL solution is water. How many milliliters of the solution is water?

Identify the unknown (define the variable) in the following situations. Make an estimate of the answer. Translate the situation to an equation. Solve the equation and check solution for reasonableness with your original estimate.

16. A pharmacy stocks 720 tablets on the shelf. Two thirds of these are used to fill prescriptions. How many tablets remain?

17. A pharmacist had 2 g of Drug C. He used it to prepare the following:

    8 capsules each containing 0.0325 g

    12 capsules each containing 0.015 g

    18 capsules each containing 0.0008 g

    How many grams of Drug C were left after he prepared the capsules?

18. A 45-gram tube of anti-itch cream contains 1% diphenhydramine hydrochloride. How many grams of the diphenhydramine hydrochloride does the tube contain?

19. A prescription written for penicillin VK 250 mg tablets instructs that one tablet be taken every 6 hours.
    a. How many tablets should the patient take each day?
    b. If the pharmacist dispenses 28 tablets, how long should the prescription last?

20. Pepcid® is available in 20-mg scored tablets.
    a. How many tablets should be given per dose if the dose is 30 mg?
    b. If the patient is to take one dose per day for 30 days, how many tablets should be dispensed?

21. Zyrtec® is available in scored 10-mg tablets. A patient takes 5 mg daily for 30 days. How many tablets are needed?

22. Mr. Blue takes one 37.5 mg Effexor® tablet twice a day for 14 days.
    a. How many tablets are taken in the 14 days?
    b. How many milligrams of Effexor® are taken over the 14 days?

23. On Monday, Ivan Aik filled his prescription for 75 Vicodin® 500-mg tablets. He takes them as needed for pain, up to eight tablets per day. By Sunday morning (6 days later), 3/5 of the original 75 tablets are left.
    a. How many are left?
    b. How many Vicodin® tablets did Ivan take?
    c. If Ivan took the same number of tablets each day, did he take more than eight tablets per day?

24. A patient takes one 20-mg tamoxifen tablet twice daily for 30 days. How many tablets are taken each month?

25. Karl Kardyo takes warfarin 5 mg once a day for 3 months (90 days). How many milligrams of warfarin does Karl take in 3 months?

Dosing Calculations and Other Pharmacy Problems

Ratios and Proportions and How to Use Them

UNIT
4

LEARNING OBJECTIVES

1. Write a mathematical ratio from a written comparison statement.
2. Convert a ratio written as a fraction to a ratio separated by a colon.
3. Identify the known concentration of a drug when given the medication label.
4. Set up and solve an equation with a variable using the ratio and proportion method.

Introduction

Ratio is the mathematical term that describes the relationship between two numerical values, or a comparison of parts to the whole. Although this definition may sound technical, most people use ratios regularly. For example, if a shopper goes to a half-off rack in a clothing store, and finds a skirt that was originally $40, she will know the new price is only $20. The new price is half of the old, or one part ($20) as compared to the two parts of the original price ($40).

Ratio—A ratio is the relationship between two quantities.

Recognizing Ratios

Ratios are written as fractions, or as parts per the whole. A colon may be used to separate the two numbers in the ratio when it is written as parts per the whole. In pharmacy, when a ratio that describes a medication concentration is written as 1:x, where x is any number, it is called a **ratio strength**. Since a percent can be written as a fraction, percents are also a kind of ratio. Ratios are often used in pharmacy to describe concentrations in compounding and in dosing calculations. In other pharmacy applications, ratios may describe the amount of one ingredient mixed in a combination of ingredients. This usage is common in compounding.

Ratio Strength—A ratio that describes a medication concentration, written as 1:x, where x is any number.

NUMBERS AT WORK
Ratios are commonly used in compounding and can be written in different ways. Understanding these differences can ensure accuracy and reduce errors.

The examples below show different ways the same ratio may be written and how they would be read.

EXAMPLE

A. ½, 1:2

B. 1/10, 1:10

C. 10:100, 10%

SOLUTION ···

Read as:

A. One half, one part per 2 parts, or one to two

B. One tenth, one part per 10 parts, or one to ten

C. 10 to 100, or 10 parts per 100, or 10 percent

When describing very small quantities of a substance that is a part of some whole, the abbreviation PPM may be used. This is another type of ratio and refers to parts per million. Ratios comparing parts per million are commonly used to describe pollutants, such as very small quantities of toxic substances in air or water.

Practice with ratios

A good grasp of how ratios are used in pharmacy is so important some extra practice is worthwhile. Keep in mind that as with fractions, the same ratio can be written in many different ways. Look at some everyday examples with which you might be familiar, below.

EXAMPLE

Your father keeps meticulous records of the miles he drives and the gas he uses. He expects you to record the miles driven and amount of gas used to fill the tank if you need gas when you borrow his car. At the gas pump, you see that filling the tank required 10.6 gallons and by the odometer you can tell that the car has been driven for 477 miles since the tank was last filled. Write a ratio that shows miles per gallon of gas used.

SOLUTION ···

The desired answer is miles per gallon. Since a fraction bar is read as "per," you can set up the ratio as a fraction. When converting a ratio from a verbal to a mathematical statement, order is important. Notice that miles are written on top and gallons below the fraction bar. Dividing both numerator and denominator by 10.6 reduces the ratio to miles per one gallon.

$$\frac{477 \text{ miles}}{10.6 \text{ gallons}} = \frac{45 \text{ miles}}{1 \text{ gal}}$$

EXAMPLE

Bactrim® DS is available as a tablet that contains trimethoprim 160 mg and sulfamethoxazole 800 mg in each tablet. What is the ratio of trimethoprim to sulfamethoxazole?

SOLUTION ···

As previously described, a ratio can be written as a fraction or divided by a colon.

trimethoprim 160 mg: sulfamethoxazole 800 mg

or

160 mg trimethoprim / 800 mg sulfamethoxazole

Since the problem asks for the ratio of trimethoprim to sulfamethoxazole, we use trimethoprim as our standard for comparison in this ratio. Reduce the ratio by dividing numerator and denominator by 160, thereby reducing the trimethoprim in the expression to 1.

1:5 is the ratio strength of trimethoprim to sulfamethoxazole in each Bactrim DS tablet

or

1 mg trimethoprim/5 mg sulfamethoxazole in each Bactrim DS tablet

Drug strengths and concentrations as ratios

Drug manufacturers are required to label prescription drugs with the strength of the individual tablet or capsule or the concentration of liquid or semisolid preparations such as ointments. Medication strengths can be written as a ratio. For example, a 10-mg enalapril tablet contains 10 mg/tablet and promethazine for injection contains 25 mg/mL.

Unlike use of solid drug formulations (tablets or capsules), the advantage of using a liquid medication is the dosing flexibility. The label of a liquid or semisolid preparation usually shows concentration of medication per mL, per 5 mL, or per vial. The volume required for each dose is calculated based on the concentration of the product and the dose ordered. Look at the following labels to see if you can find the concentration for each product pictured.

EXAMPLES

Write the drug strengths or concentrations found on the following labels as ratios.

A. Amoxicillin pediatric drops

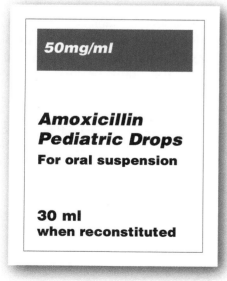

50mg/ml

Amoxicillin Pediatric Drops
For oral suspension

30 ml
when reconstituted

B. Flumazenil Injection

C. Carboplatin for injection

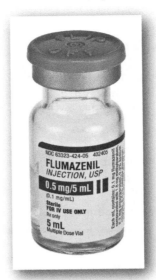

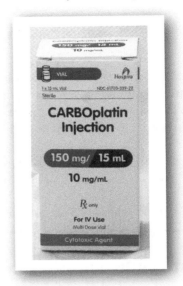

Source: Reprinted with permission of APP Pharmaceuticals.

Source: Reprinted with permission of Hospira, Inc.

SOLUTIONS

A. Amoxicillin pediatric drops labeling shows the concentration as 50 mg/ per mL after the product is reconstituted.

B. The labeling for flumazenil shows both the concentration per mL (0.1 mg/ mL) and the concentration per 5 mL, the amount in the vial (0.5 mg/5 mL).

C. Carboplatin injection lists the concentration as 150 mg/15 mL and as 10 mg/mL.

Proportion Equations

In the previous section a ratio was defined as a mathematical statement that compares one value to another. In the example of the Bactrim® DS tablets, the contents of one tablet contained 160 mg trimethoprim per 800 mg sulfamethoxazole. The ratio of trimethoprim to sulfamethoxazole in Bactrim® DS tablets never changes, whether you consider one tablet, multiple tablets, or a tiny fraction of a tablet. Notice that after this ratio was reduced, it read 1 mg trimethoprim/5 mg sulfamethoxazole. The ratio for one tablet and the reduced ratio are equal and can be written as an equation.

$$\frac{160 \text{ mg trimethoprim}}{800 \text{ mg sulfamethoxazole}} = \frac{1 \text{ mg trimethoprim}}{5 \text{ mg sulfamethoxazole}}$$

This is called a **proportion equation**, which is an equation of two equal ratios. Proportion equations are useful in pharmacy because a known ratio can be used to solve for an unknown value. This is called the ratio and proportion method of solving for an unknown.

Proportion Equation—An equation of two equal ratios.

EXAMPLE

Tobramycin injection is provided as a sterile solution of 80 mg tobramycin in 2 mL of solution.

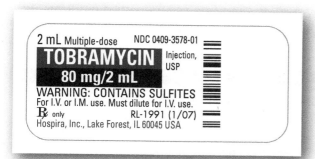

Source: Reprinted with permission of Hospira, Inc.

You receive the following drug order for Anita Schotz, a hospitalized patient with a serious infection:

> tobramycin 120 mg
> IVPB Q12h

You must draw up the tobramycin solution to prepare the IV piggyback bags. How much tobramycin solution will be added to each piggyback bag?

SOLUTION

The labeled concentration is 80 mg tobramycin per 2 mL solution and 120 mg is needed for each bag. The volume (in mL) that contains 120 mg tobramycin for injection is unknown. To solve for this unknown, set up a proportion equation where x = the volume of tobramycin that contains 120 mg.

$$\frac{80 \text{ mg}}{2 \text{ mL}} = \frac{120 \text{ mg}}{x}$$

To solve a proportion equation, use cross multiplication. In other words, the numerator of the left side of the equation is multiplied by the denominator of the right side of the equation and that is set equal to the numerator of the right side times the denominator of the left side.

$$\frac{80 \text{ mg}}{2 \text{ mL}} = \frac{120 \text{ mg}}{x}$$

$$x \text{ (80 mg)} = 120 \text{ mg (2 mL)}$$

Remember that to solve an equation, the unknown (in this case x) must be isolated on one side of the equation. Notice that the units (mg) cancel out on both sides of the equation.

$$\frac{x \text{ (80 mg)}}{80 \text{ mg}} = \frac{120 \text{ mg (2 mL)}}{80 \text{ mg}}$$

$$x = \frac{120 \text{ (2 mL)}}{80} = 3 \text{ mL}$$

This process may seem cumbersome for those students that were able to look at this problem and know that if 80 mg = 2 mL, then 40 mg = 1 mL, and 120 mg = 3 mL. However, as you will see, not all proportion problems are this easy to visualize. Therefore, it is essential to become very comfortable with setting up and solving this type of equation.

Practice with proportion equations

Since almost all pharmacy-related problems can be solved with this type of equation, it makes sense to look at a few more ratio and proportion problems. Try setting up and solving the equations before you look at the answers in the problems below.

EXAMPLE

Mrs. Pickles' 6-month-old baby boy Dillon has an ear infection. The pediatrician ordered amoxicillin drops (see label in Example A, above) 60 mg twice daily. What volume of amoxicillin 50 mg/mL pediatric drops will contain the 60-mg dose? Remember to estimate before you calculate.

SOLUTION ·

The label and the problem state that 1 mL of amoxicillin pediatric drops contain 50 mg. Since 1 mL contains 50 mg, then 2 mL will contain 100 mg. Therefore, you can estimate the required volume for a 60-mg dose will be just a little more than 1 mL. Set up a proportion equation with the known concentration on one side, and the desired dose on the other.

$$\frac{50 \text{ mg}}{1 \text{ mL}} = \frac{60 \text{ mg}}{?}$$

In this case (?) = an unknown volume of amoxicillin pediatric drops that contains 60 mg.

Next, cross multiply and rearrange the equation.

$$60 \text{ mg} (1 \text{ mL}) = 50 \text{ mg} (?)$$

Now, solve for the unknown by dividing both sides of the equation by 50 mg.

$$\frac{60 \text{ mg} (1 \text{ mL})}{50 \text{ mg}} = \frac{50 \text{ mg} (?)}{50 \text{ mg}}$$

1.2 mL = ? volume

The answer indicates that 1.2 mL amoxicillin pediatric drops contain 60 mg amoxicillin. Because we estimated first, we also know this answer is in the range of what was expected.

Notice that in every example of proportion equations used so far, the units in the numerators and denominators of both ratios are the same. In order to use this method, units must always be the same on both sides of the equation.

▶ TECH NOTE! ───────────────────

In order to use a proportion equation to solve for an unknown value, the units in the numerators of both ratios and the units in the denominators of both ratios must be the same.

So, what options are available to solve for an unknown (using the ratio and proportion method) when the given ratio uses different units than the desired answer? Any time you have different units in the ratios, convert to the desired units before setting up and solving the equation. Look at the following example.

EXAMPLE

Vancomycin for injection is sold in a vial that contains 1 gram vancomycin in powder form for reconstitution. In the hospital pharmacy where you work, vancomycin vials are diluted to a final concentration of 1 g/20 mL. The pharmacist asks you to make three vancomycin 650 mg IV piggyback bags. How much reconstituted vancomycin solution will you add to each bag?

SOLUTION

The reconstituted vancomycin solution contains 1 g/20 mL, but the question asks for the volume that contains 650 mg. If you are not paying attention to the units as you set up the ratios, you might set up the proportion equation with grams in the numerator on the left side and milligrams in the numerator on the right. This is not a valid proportion equation.

$$\cancel{1g\,/20\,mL = 650\,mg/x}$$

If the units are tracked when solving the equation, the remaining units that don't cancel will be a clue that there is an error. The way to proceed with this problem is to convert grams to milligrams, then set up the ratio and solve.

$$1 \text{ gram} = 1000 \text{ mg}$$
$$1000 \text{ mg}/20 \text{ mL} = 650 \text{ mg}/x$$
$$\frac{650 \cancel{\text{ mg}} (20 \text{ mL})}{1000 \cancel{\text{ mg}}} = \frac{1000 \cancel{\text{ mg}} (x)}{1000 \cancel{\text{ mg}}}$$
$$13 \text{ mL} = x$$

Sometimes ratios are expressed with a colon separating the two values instead of a fraction bar.

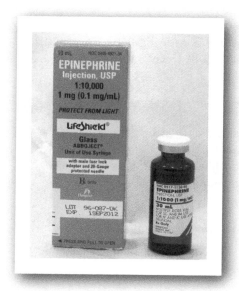

Epinephrine 1:10,000 and 1:1000. *Source:* Reprinted with permission of Hospira, Inc., and American Regent, Inc.

Labeling for epinephrine, for instance, is often expressed in this fashion. When working with a proportion equation expressed this way there are two choices. Either change the expression to the kind of ratio separated with a fraction bar, being careful to insert the correct units, or learn the following way of solving this type of ratio and proportion equation.

EXAMPLE

A nurse calls to say she has 1 mL of a 1:1000 solution (1 gram per 1000 mL) of epinephrine. She needs to give a patient 0.6 mg epinephrine subcutaneously. How much of the solution should she administer?

SOLUTION

First convert grams to mg in the known ratio so that you will have the same units in each ratio.

1 gram = 1000 mg, so the known ratio will read 1000:1000
The unknown ratio is set up like this:
0.6:x

To set up a proportion equation using this type of ratio, a double colon is used in place of an equal sign. The outer numbers in the equation are called the "extremes" and the inner numbers are called the "means."

$$1000:1000 :: 0.6:x$$

Means / Extremes

When a proportion equation is set up in this manner, the product of the means is equal to the product of the extremes. To solve, the equation is rewritten as follows:

$$1000 \text{ mg } (x) = 1000 \text{ mL } (0.6 \text{ mg})$$
$$x = \frac{1000 \text{ mL } (0.6 \text{ mg})}{1000 \text{ mg}}$$
$$x = 0.6 \text{ mL}$$

Proportion equations can also be used when converting between systems of measurement. The conversion factor becomes the "known" ratio. Look at the example below.

EXAMPLE

Mrs. Shoop brings in a prescription for her 4-year-old son, Campbell. He is a new patient, and you are assigned to create a patient profile for him. Campbell weighs 38 pounds, but the patient profile requires the weight in kilograms. How will you convert his weight in pounds to kg?

SOLUTION

The conversion factor of 2.2 lb/kg is the known ratio. Campbell's weight in pounds divided by the unknown (x) becomes the other ratio in the proportion equation.

$$\frac{38 \text{ lb}}{x} = \frac{2.2 \text{ lb}}{1 \text{ kg}}$$

$$2.2 \text{ lb } (x) = 38 \text{ lb } (1 \text{ kg})$$

$$x = \frac{38 \text{ lb } (1 \text{ kg})}{2.2 \text{ lb}}$$

$$x = 17.3 \text{ kg}$$

The ratio and proportion method for solving problems is invaluable in pharmacy. It can be used for calculating doses, making conversions between systems of measurements and in compounding. Table 9-1 summarizes what you have learned about ratio and proportion problems. Now, put in some time working practice problems so that you can master this important method.

Table 9-1. Steps in Solving a Ratio and Proportion Equation

1. Find your known ratio.
2. Set up the ratio with the unknown.
3. Check to make sure the units in the numerators are the same in both ratios, and that the units in the denominators are the same.
4. Estimate your answer.
5. Solve by cross multiplying, and compare your answer with your estimate.

Practice Problems

1. Write the following statements as ratios:
   a. Many potato salad recipes call for 6 cups of peeled and chopped potatoes for 8 servings of potato salad.
   b. Jennifer drives 475 miles on 10.5 gallons of gas in her new Prius.
   c. Mylanta suspension costs $6.99 for 12 oz.
   d. There are 900 calories in a double cheeseburger.

2. Write the following statements as ratios, using a colon to separate the values:
   a. 1 gram per 10,000 mL
   b. 3 grams per 100 mL
   c. 1 part of vinegar to 3 parts of olive oil

3. Write the following ratios as fractions:
   a. 3:4
   b. 1:10
   c. 9:1000
   d. 2:3

4. Write the following dosage strengths as ratios:
   a. Tetracycline 250-mg capsule
   b. Phenobarbital 20 mg in 5 milliliters
   c. Amikacin 250 mg per mL
   d. 10-mg enalapril tablet

5. On the following drug labels, find the drug strength per mL.
   a.

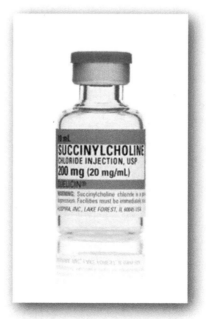

Source: Reprinted with permission of Hospira, Inc.

b.

Solu-Medrol® label:

For IM or IV use
Single-Dose Vial
Protect from light.
DOSAGE AND USE: See accompanying prescribing information.
* Each mL (when mixed) contains methylprednisolone sodium succinate equivalent to methylprednisolone 40 mg. Lyophilized in container.
Distributed by Pharmacia & Upjohn Co
Division of Pfizer Inc, NY, NY 10017

Rx only   1 mL Act-O-Vial® NDC 0009-0039-30

Solu-Medrol®
methylprednisolone sodium succinate for injection, USP

40 mg*

Preservative-Free

LOT/EXP   10751900   N 03 0009-0039-30-1   FP0 - RSS 7 Mil

Source: Reprinted with permission of Pfizer, Inc.

UNIT
4

6. When solving a ratio and proportion equation, make sure the _____ are the same in the numerator and denominator of each ratio.

7. A vial of furosemide for injection contains 40 mg/4 mL. What volume of furosemide for injection contains 10 mg?

8. Paul, the P.T., needs to add 600 mg of vancomycin to an IVPB bag. When reconstituted, the vancomycin vial will contain 1 g/10 mL. What volume of reconstituted vancomycin solution will Paul draw up in the syringe in order to add the required 600 mg?

9. Epinephrine is available in a 1:1000 solution and a 1:10,000 solution.
   a. Which product contains more epinephrine per mL?
   b. How many mg of epinephrine are in 10 mL of a 1:10,000 solution?

10. An IVPB order calls for amikacin 350 mg. The pharmacy stocks 500-mg vials that contain 2 mL. What volume of this solution will provide the needed 350 mg?

11. The ABC pharmacy in the pediatrics clinic carries erythromycin ethyl succinate suspension in a concentration of 400 mg/5 mL. Dr. Darlene Bebe ordered a dose of 300 mg Q6 hours and wants a 10-day supply for her patient.
    a. What volume of the suspension contains 300 mg erythromycin ethyl succinate?
    b. Should the pharmacy dispense the 100-mL bottle or the 200-mL bottle to provide enough for 10 days?

12. Normal saline solution contains 0.9 g sodium chloride in 100 mL. How much sodium chloride is contained in 250 mL normal saline?

13. Phenytoin oral suspension contains 125 mg of the drug in 5 mL. The physician orders 250 mg to be given every 12 hours.
    a. What volume of the suspension will the patient receive per dose?
    b. When taken according to the directions, how many mL will the patient receive in a day?
    c. How long will an 8 fl oz bottle last?

14. Mia Cord brings in a prescription for carvedilol. She is to take 9.75 mg twice daily for early heart failure and elevated blood pressure. Carvedilol is available in strengths of 3.25 mg and 6.5 mg.
    a. Which strength would you choose to fill this prescription and why?
    b. How will the directions for dosing read?

15. Solve the following proportion equations:
    a. $1:10,000 :: 5:x$
    b. $1 \text{ gram}/10 \text{ mL} = x/350 \text{ mL}$
    c. $500 \text{ mcg}/2 \text{ mL} = 750 \text{ mcg}/x$
    d. $3:18 :: x:162$

16. Drug Y 292.5 grams is the active ingredient used to make 130,000 tablets. What is the strength, in milligrams, of one tablet?

17. A 20-mL multidose vial of vaccine costs $475. One dose of vaccine is 0.5 mL.
    a. How many people can be vaccinated with one vial?
    b. What is the cost per dose of vaccine?

18. Maxeton Compounding Pharmacy's special "Baby's Bottom" diaper ointment contains 10 grams of zinc oxide and 30 mL of antacid in every 100 grams of ointment. The pharmacist at Maxeton Pharmacy asks Howie Dewitt, the new technician, to make one pound of the diaper ointment.
    a. How many grams of ointment are in 1 pound?
    b. How much zinc oxide will Howie weigh out for one pound of ointment?
    c. How much antacid suspension will Howie measure for the ointment?

19. You are planning a pizza party for the pharmacy department. On average, each person usually eats three slices of pizza, and a large pie contains 12 slices. There are 17 pharmacists and technicians coming. How many large pizzas should you order to make sure there is enough for 3 slices each?

20. The total weight of 100 alprazolam 0.5-mg tablets is 3.75 grams. What is the ratio of active ingredient to filler in 100 tablets?

21. Deanna, the dietician, is talking to Betty Baker, recently diagnosed with diabetes, about her diet. Betty loves to make apple pies. Deanna says the calories in a 9-inch apple pie come from 260 g carbohydrates (from apples, sugar, and flour) and 110 g fat. The entire pie contains 2030 calories.
    a. If the pie is divided in 8 equal pieces, how many calories are in 3 pieces?
    b. There are 1040 calories provided by the 260 g of carbohydrates in the whole pie. How many calories does 1 gram of carbohydrate provide?
    c. If the remaining calories come from 110 grams of fat, how many calories are derived from 1 gram of fat?

22. The dermatologist in Our Town Pharmacy has a special formula for erythromycin 2% gel. The formula contains:

Erythromycin	2 g
Hydroxypropyl cellulose	2 g
Ethyl alcohol 70% qs	100 mL

You are asked to make up a pint of the gel.

a. How much erythromycin is needed to make 1 pint?

b. How much hydroxypropyl cellulose is needed to make 1 pint?

23. **Our Town Pharmacy is running out of the ingredients for the formulation in Problem 22. The pharmacist asks you to order erythromycin and hydroxypropyl cellulose to make a 3-month's supply of the erythromycin 2% gel. She says that the average amount compounded in 1 month is 2.5 liters. The powder is available in 500-g containers and the hydroxypropyl cellulose is available in 1-pound containers. How many containers of each will you order?**

24. **Peter Ivanakoff has a cold. He decides to purchase a bottle of cough syrup that contains guaifenesin 200 mg and pseudoephedrine 40 mg in 5 mL.**

a. How much guaifenesin and pseudoephedrine are contained in 8 fluid ounces of the syrup?

b. If the patient takes 10 mL of the syrup three times a day, how many days will an 8-fluid ounce bottle last?

25. **Riley Quick, C.Ph.T., and Nita Gallop, C.Ph.T., have decided to see who is fastest at counting and pouring medication for prescriptions. Nita does the counting and pouring for 43 prescriptions in 3.5 hours. How many prescriptions will Riley need to prepare in his 7.5-hour shift to beat Nita?**

CHAPTER 10

Calculating Drug Doses

LEARNING OBJECTIVES

1. Define the terms *dose* and *dosing regimen*.
2. Convert a given dose to needed volume of solution or number of tablets.
3. Calculate a dose based on weight.
4. Calculate a dose based on body surface area.
5. Explain how sliding scale insulin orders are used.

UNIT 4

Dose—A specified quantity of a therapeutic agent, such as a drug or medicine, prescribed to be taken at one time or at stated intervals.

Dosing Regimen—The expected amount of medication prescribed per time unit and duration of dosing.

Introduction

Dosing calculations are some of the most common pharmacy math problems the pharmacy technician will face in practice. A **dose** is the amount of medication to be taken by the patient at a given time and a **dosing regimen** is the prescribed amount of medication with the frequency and duration of the therapy included. Prescribers usually specify the amount of a single dose in a drug order, so little in the way of calculations is likely to be needed, unless a volume of liquid medication or number of tablets needs to be determined. In some cases, the prescriber will provide a dose based on weight, body surface area, or other criteria. Pharmacy technicians are expected to know how to make these initial dosing calculations, or to provide a double check for the pharmacist.

Common Dosing Problems

You have already been introduced to some basic dosage calculation problems. Calculations are required when the ordered dose does not exactly match available strengths of tablets or capsules, when technicians are compounding sterile solutions where the volume of medication is more or less than one vial, and when a liquid formulation is ordered that will require a patient to measure out a to-be-determined volume of medication. When liquids are prescribed to outpatients, the volume of medication must be indicated on the label in order for the dose to be correctly administered. You can either use a ratio and proportion equation or dimensional analysis to solve these basic dosing problems. Look over the following examples for a quick review.

EXAMPLE

Pharmacy technician Lottie Warrick receives a prescription for hydrochlorothiazide 37.5 mg to be administered once daily in the morning. The pharmacy has hydrochlorothiazide 25 mg per tablet available. How should the patient be instructed to take this medication?

SOLUTION ···

To solve this problem using the ratio and proportion method, determine what the known ratio is and then set up the unknown ratio for the proportion equation.

Known ratio: 25 mg/tablet; unknown ratio: 37.5 mg/x. Therefore your proportion equation will look like this:

$$\frac{25 \text{ mg}}{\text{tablet}} = \frac{37.5 \text{ mg}}{x}$$

$$37.5 \text{ mg (tablet)} = 25 \text{ mg } (x)$$

$$x = \frac{37.5 \text{ mg (tablet)}}{25 \text{ mg}}$$

$$x = 1.5 \text{ tablets}$$

The patient will be instructed to take 1½ tablets (37.5 mg) once daily in the morning. Remember to include both the number of tablets and the dose in milligrams on the label for clarity.

Dimensional analysis is another useful technique for calculating dosages. In dosage problems, first determine what units the answer should have. Then multiply by a conversion ratio equal to 1 of the desired units. This ratio is determined from information in a conversion table or information on the medication label.

EXAMPLE

A physician orders a 50-mg dose of medication. The pharmacy stocks 25-mg tablets. How many tablets should be administered?

SOLUTION ···

The desired unit is "tablets."
Next, find a conversion ratio equal to 1.

$$1 \text{ tablet} = 25 \text{ mg}$$

$$\frac{1 \text{ tablet}}{25 \text{ mg}} = \frac{25 \text{ mg}}{25 \text{ mg}}$$

$$\frac{1 \text{ tablet}}{25 \text{ mg}} = 1$$

Now, use this conversion ratio to solve the problem.

$$50 \text{ mg} \left(\frac{1 \text{ tablet}}{25 \text{ mg}} \right) = 2 \text{ tablets}$$

EXAMPLE

A patient is to take 0.75 mL of medication. The medication is labeled as 10 mg per mL. How many milligrams will the patient receive?

SOLUTION

The desired units are milligrams. The information on the label states that there are 10 mg/mL. Therefore:

$$0.75 \text{ mL} \left(\frac{10 \text{ mg}}{\text{mL}} \right) = 7.5 \text{ mg}$$

EXAMPLE

A patient that weighs 40.9 kg is to receive Medication M tablets in a dose of 15 mg/kg. What will the dose be?

SOLUTION

The answer should be in milligrams.

$$40.9 \text{ kg} \times \frac{15 \text{ mg}}{\text{kg}} = 613.5 \text{ mg}$$

Undoubtedly, in order to be measured, a drug dose of 613.5 mg will be rounded. How the dose is rounded would depend on the available formulation or concentration of the drug. Medication M is a 150-mg tablet, so in this example the dose would be rounded to 600 mg.

EXAMPLE

Since Medication M is supplied as 150-mg tablets, how many tablets should be given for the 600-mg dose?

SOLUTION

The correct answer will be in units of "tablets."

$$1 \text{ tablet} = 150 \text{ mg}$$

$$\frac{1 \text{ tablet}}{150 \text{ mg}} = 1$$

$$600 \text{ mg} \left(\frac{1 \text{ tablet}}{150 \text{ mg}} \right) = 4 \text{ tablets}$$

EXAMPLE

You receive the following drug order for Buster Hart:

Digoxin 0.25 mg IVP daily

The label on the digoxin for injection indicates the ampule contains 500 mcg digoxin/2 mL. What volume will the nurse draw into a syringe to deliver 0.25 mg of digoxin?

SOLUTION

You can use dimensional analysis or a proportion equation to solve this problem. The equation below represents the dimensional analysis method. Start by canceling units, and then perform the mathematical operation. Your answer should be in mL.

$$0.25 \text{ mg digoxin} \times \frac{2 \text{ mL}}{500 \text{ mcg}} \times \frac{1000 \text{ mcg}}{\text{mg}} =$$

$$\frac{0.25 \times 2 \text{ mL} \times 1000}{500} = 1 \text{ mL}$$

Alternatively, using the ratio and proportion method looks like this:

$$500 \text{ mcg} = 0.5 \text{ mg}$$
$$0.5 \text{ mg}/2 \text{ mL} = 0.25 \text{ mg}/x$$
$$0.5 \text{ mg} (x) = 2 \text{ mL} (0.25 \text{ mg})$$
$$x = \frac{2 \text{ mL} (0.25 \text{ mg})}{0.5 \text{ mg}}$$
$$x = 1 \text{ mL}$$

Dosing Based on Body Weight

In normal adults, drugs are often dosed with a one size fits all approach. However, there are situations when the standard adult dose does not work. For example, adults with kidney failure often require a reduced dose of certain drugs. In order to achieve more appropriate dosing, some drugs are dosed based on body weight. Weight-based dosing is not too common in adults, but it is the standard of practice in infants, children and adolescents. The use of weight-based dosing requires that the technician be comfortable converting body weight from pounds to kilograms and then calculating the dose.

NUMBERS AT WORK
Knowing the calculation to convert body weight in pounds to kilograms is critical to weight-based dosing in pediatric patients.

EXAMPLE

The following drug order is sent to the hospital pharmacy where you work. How much gentamicin will the patient receive (see Figure 10-1)?

Figure 10-1. A typical weight-based drug order seen in a hospital.

4/23/12	Gentamicin 3 mg/kg x 1 dose
	IVPB, then pharmacist to
	manage gentamicin dosing x 10
	days for pneumonia. Patient
	weighs 167 lb.

SOLUTION

The first step in finding the answer to this problem is to convert the patient's weight in pounds to the correct weight in kilograms. As you recall, the conversion factor for pounds to kilograms is 2.2 lb/kilogram. The proportion equation will look like this:

$$2.2 \text{ lb/kilogram} = 167 \text{ lb}/x$$
$$x = \frac{167 \text{ (kg)}}{2.2}$$
$$x = 75.9 \text{ kg}$$

To determine the one-time IVPB dose of gentamicin, multiply the patient's weight in kilograms by the weight-based dose as follows:

$$75.9 \text{ kg} \times 3 \text{ mg/kg} = 227.7 \text{ mg}$$

Gentamicin solution is available in a concentration of 40 mg/mL, so 227.7 mg is not going to be measurable in the syringes available for this task. Most pharmacists would round this dose to 230 mg.

EXAMPLE

What volume will the technician draw up in the syringe to make a 230-mg IVPB bag?

SOLUTION

Gentamicin for injection in stock contains 40 mg/mL.

$$40 \text{ mg/1 mL} = 230 \text{ mg}/x$$
$$x = \frac{230 \text{ (1 mL)}}{40} = 5.75 \text{ mL gentamicin injection}$$

Caring for pediatric patients

Pediatric patients come in all sizes, from tiny, premature newborns to husky, fully grown, 18-year-old football players. It is not at all uncommon to find patients that weigh from 1 kg (2.2 pounds) to 100 kg (220 pounds) in any pediatric specialty hospital on any given day. Because of the potential for huge differences in doses, pharmacists and pharmacy technicians must be particularly vigilant when it comes to calculating drug doses in pediatric patients.

In order to accurately calculate a drug dose based on body weight, the weight must be correct. Technicians working in a pediatric setting should always check the child's age against the weight provided in the chart or patient profile to see if the weight makes sense. An easy to remember, rough guideline is helpful when judging whether a child's recorded weight makes sense. Between 1 and 2 years of age, a child's weight in pounds is normally in the teens to twenties, a child of 3 years weighs in the thirties (pounds), a child of 4 weighs in the forties. From 4 or 5 years of age to around age 10, growth is more gradual. A typical 10-year-old boy or girl usually weighs in the 70–90 pound range. With adolescence there is no easy way to predict heights and weights. But, if you can keep these rough approximations in mind, you may be able to recognize when to double check listed weights and avoid disastrous dosing errors. Look at the following problem.

EXAMPLE

Vera Wong is a 4.5-year-old girl admitted to a pediatric hospital to undergo treatment for chronic ear infection and chronic mastoiditis. There are drug orders for IV antibiotics based on her weight, which is listed as 42 kg. Do you think it is appropriate to follow through with making the IV antibiotic as ordered?

SOLUTION

Unless you are very familiar with what 42 kg looks like, convert this weight to pounds to help you decide whether to ask the pharmacist to verify the weight before making the IV antibiotics.

$$42 \text{ kg} \times 2.2 \text{ lb/kg} = 92.4 \text{ lb}$$

Even with our nationwide childhood obesity problem, it is highly unlikely that a 4.5-year-old would weigh 92.4 pounds. The odds are that this weight is erroneous and clearly worth rechecking. In this scenario what may have happened is the weight in pounds was entered in the computer as though it was the weight in kilograms. This type of error sometimes happens in the hospital setting. Always check weight calculations by looking at the answer to see if it makes sense. If the number obtained in a conversion to kilograms is larger than the same weight in pounds, there is an error.

> **TECH NOTE!**
>
> *A patient's weight in kilograms will always be a smaller number (less than half) than the patient's weight in pounds.*

Weight-based dosing orders may be written as mg/kg/dose or mg/kg/day. Orders written as a total daily dose will include instructions that the total be divided into a given number of doses. In a pediatric population, where errors can be devastating, the order should clearly distinguish between these two possibilities. If there is any doubt, verify your interpretation with the pharmacist.

EXAMPLE

Haywood Yaczecht, pharmacy technician at Happy Valley Children's hospital, receives the following order:

Furosemide solution 2 mg/kg, Q6h

Haywood is not sure whether this is supposed to be a daily dose divided into q6h doses or if this is the amount the prescriber wants to be given each dose. What should he do?

SOLUTION

Because the prescriber has included a comma after the dose and has not indicated whether this is a single dose or a total daily dose, this order is ambiguous. Haywood needs to clarify this order with the pharmacist before proceeding. If this order is intended as the amount to be given per dose it is more correctly written:

Furosemide solution 2 mg/kg/dose Q6h

A daily, weight-based order would be appropriately written:

Furosemide solution 2 mg/kg/day in four divided doses

EXAMPLE

The pharmacist determines that the order is intended to be given per dose. The 3-year-old child for whom the furosemide is ordered weighs 14 kg. How many milligrams of furosemide will he receive per dose?

SOLUTION ···

14 kg × 2 mg/kg/dose = 28 mg furosemide per dose

Dosing Based on Body Surface Area

Body surface area (BSA) is the measured or calculated area of the human body. An individual's body surface area is based on height and weight and is expressed in meters squared (m²). Use of body surface area for drug dosing was initially introduced in clinical trials of toxic drugs so researchers could extrapolate a safe starting dose for humans based on toxicity studies done in animals. It is felt to be a safer basis for dosing because BSA is less affected by obesity. Most cancer chemotherapy drugs are dosed based on body surface area.

Body Surface Area—The measured or calculated surface area of the human body, expressed in meters squared.

Body surface area nomograms

While there are many formulas to calculate body surface area, most pharmacies use a nomogram, like the ones shown in Figures 10-2 and 10-3.

Notice that there are two nomograms; one used to determine BSA in children and one used in adults. To find the body service area, mark the patient's height on line A and weight on line C. Using a straight edge to connect the two points, read the body surface area on line B. Look at the following example to try using the nomograms.

EXAMPLE

The oncologist has ordered a one-time IV dose of methotrexate 100 mg/m² for a 4-year-old boy with acute lymphocytic leukemia. He is 41 inches tall and weighs 39 pounds. What is his body surface area? What will the dose of methotrexate be?

SOLUTION ···

On the pediatric nomogram, mark a dot at 41 inches (line A) and 39 pounds (line B). Draw a straight line through the two points. The body surface area is 0.75 m². The dose will be calculated as follows:

100 mg/m² × 0.75 m² = 75 mg

Figure 10-2. Body surface area nomogram for pediatric patients.

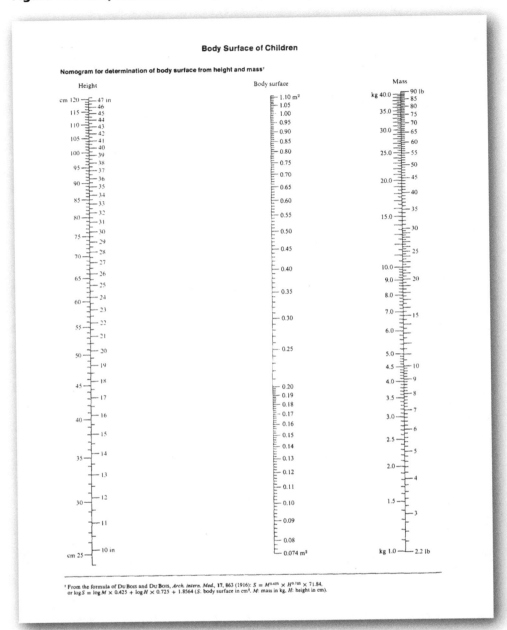

Source: Reprinted with permission from *Geigy Scientific Tables*. Vol. 1. 8th ed. Lentner C, ed. Basle, Switzerland: CIBA-GEIGY Limited; 1993:226.

Drug Doses Measured in International Units

Several important drugs are measured in international units instead of metric weight. An **international unit** measures biological activity or effect of a substance. Insulin, a hormone used to treat diabetes, and heparin, an anticoagulant, are both measured in units.

International Unit—An internationally agreed upon amount of a substance, based on its biological activity.

Figure 10-3. Body surface area for adult patients.

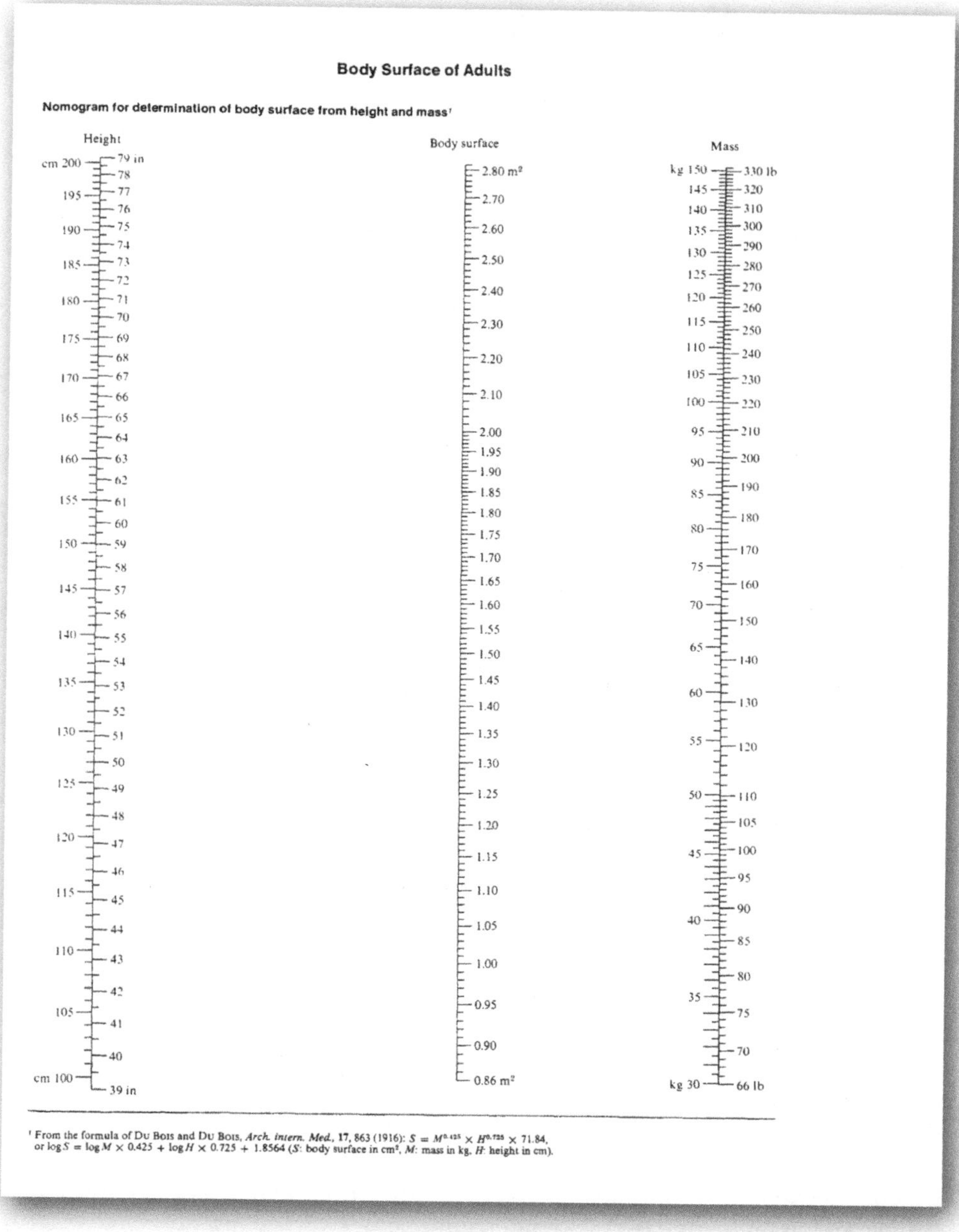
Body Surface of Adults
Nomogram for determination of body surface from height and mass[1]
Height
cm 200
79 in
cm 100
39 in
Body surface
2.80 m²
0.86 m²
Mass
kg 150
330 lb
kg 30
66 lb
[1] From the formula of Du Bois and Du Bois, Arch. intern. Med., 17, 863 (1916): S = M^0.425 × H^0.725 × 71.84, or log S = log M × 0.425 + log H × 0.725 + 1.8564 (S: body surface in cm², M: mass in kg, H: height in cm).

Source: Reprinted with permission from *Geigy Scientific Tables*. Vol. 1. 8th ed. Lentner C, ed. Basle, Switzerland: CIBA-GEIGY Limited; 1993:226.

TECH NOTE!

No matter how drug doses are being measured, a ratio and a proportion equation can still be used to solve for an unknown.

UNIT 4

Look at the dosing of heparin to illustrate this concept in the example below.

Will B. Klotz is a salesman who recently returned home from a long road trip. He arrives at the hospital in an ambulance with shortness of breath and chest pain. The E.R. physician believes Will has a pulmonary embolism, and he orders a 50 units/kg body weight loading dose of heparin. Will weighs 168 pounds. The heparin you have in the pharmacy is 5000 units per mL. How many units of heparin will he receive? What volume of heparin 5000 units/mL will the nurse draw up to administer the dose?

SOLUTION ··

First, convert Will's weight to kilograms.

$$\frac{1 \text{ kg}}{2.2 \text{ lb}} \times 168 \text{ lb} = 76.4 \text{ kg}$$

Now, round his weight to the nearest whole kilogram, and calculate the dose of heparin.

$$76 \text{ kg} \times 50 \text{ units/kg} = 3800 \text{ units}$$

Will's heparin dose is 3800 units. To determine the volume of heparin, use the ratio and proportion method to solve.

$$\frac{5000 \text{ units}}{\text{mL}} = \frac{3800 \text{ units}}{x}$$

$$5000 \text{ units } (x) = 3800 \text{ units (mL)}$$

$$x = \frac{3800 \text{ units (mL)}}{5000 \text{ units}}$$

$x = 0.76$ mL of heparin 5,000 units/mL will deliver the necessary dose

Measuring and calculating insulin doses

Although there are a variety of different types of insulin on the market, they are all measured in units. For insulin, a unit is an internationally agreed upon measure that was determined based on its ability to reduce blood glucose by a specified amount. All types of insulin now contain 100 units of insulin/mL, which is referred to as U-100 insulin (see Figure 10-4). Insulin is measured in syringes that are marked in units for easier patient dosing.

Current practices in diabetes management usually include treatment with long-acting insulin for basal or background sugar requirements and rapid-acting insulin for mealtime sugar elevations. Sometimes patients have to calculate additional doses of rapid acting insulin to give when their blood sugar is elevated before meals. These dosing calculations are based on rough estimates of expected insulin activity in a patient. Look at the following example to see how additional dose calculations are made.

Sue Sweet uses 4 units of NovoLog® insulin before meals and adds additional units if her blood sugar is higher than her target of 120 mg/dL. When she tested her glucose level before lunch, she found that her level was 220 mg/dL. Sue's physician instructed her to give 1 extra unit of insulin for every 50 mg/dL above the target glucose level. How much NovoLog® should Sue inject?

SOLUTION ···

Calculate the insulin requirement by finding the difference between the target and actual blood sugar levels first.

$$220 \text{ mg/dL} - 120 \text{ mg/dL} = 100 \text{ mg/dL}$$

Sue is to give 1 extra unit of insulin per 50 mg/dL sugar excess.

$$\frac{1 \text{ unit}}{50 \text{ mg/dL}} = \frac{x}{100 \text{ mg/dL excess}}$$

$$x \,(50 \text{ mg/dL}) = 1 \text{ unit } (100 \text{ mg/dL excess})$$

$$x = 2 \text{ units}$$

So, Sue will give herself her usual 4 units of insulin plus 2 additional units, for a total lunchtime dose of 6 units.

This kind of dosing, where additional insulin is given based on blood sugar results, is often referred to as "sliding scale" dosing. Technicians need to understand this variable kind of dosing so that they will correctly interpret prescriptions and refer patient questions appropriately.

Figure 10-4. Two different types of insulin. All insulin is sold in 100 units/mL concentration.

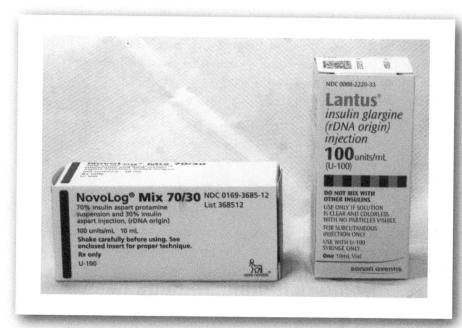

Source (left): Reprinted with permission of Novo Nordisk Inc., and (right) with permission by Sanofi US.

Practice Problems

1. A drug order from the nursing home your pharmacy services reads "venlafaxine 56.25 mg p.o. BID." The pharmacy carries 37.5-mg tablets and 75-mg tablets.
   a. What strength tablets will you use to fill this order and why?
   b. How many tablets will the patient take per dose?

2. A drug order for Tammy Taylor, a 2-year-old, reads ondansetron 0.15 mg/kg IV push to be given as a premedication before chemotherapy. Tammy weighs 25 pounds. The pharmacy stocks ondansetron injection 4 mg/2 mL.
   a. What is Tammy's weight in kg?
   b. What is the dose of ondansetron she will receive?
   c. What volume of ondansetron solution contains this dose?

3. Hedda Aiken is an 18-month-old admitted to the pediatric hospital with meningitis. The admitting physician orders Rocephin®, 80 mg/kg/day, in two divided doses. Hedda weighs 19 pounds.
   a. What is Hedda's weight in kg?
   b. How many milligrams of Rocephin® will Hedda receive?
   c. The hospital carries Rocephin® in a ready-to-use formulation that contains 1 gram in 50 mL. What volume will you draw up to fill Hedda's order?

4. You receive a prescription for azithromycin suspension that contains 200 mg/5 mL when reconstituted. The physician wants the patient to receive 400 mg on the first day and 200 mg daily for the next 4 days.
   a. How many mL of suspension will the patient take with the first dose?
   b. What volume will the patient take each day thereafter?
   c. This product is available in 15-mL, 22.5-mL, and 30-mL sizes. Which size will last for the whole 5-day course?

5. You are making IVPB solutions. There are three different orders for gentamicin piggybacks. You have available a 30-mL vial of gentamicin 40 mg/mL.
   a. What volume of gentamicin solution will you draw up in a syringe to make a 60-mg IVPB?
   b. What volume of gentamicin do you need to make a 100-mg piggyback bag?
   c. After making two 60-mg doses, one 100-mg dose, and three 80-mg doses, how much gentamicin will be left in the vial?

6. A female patient with a yeast infection comes to the pharmacy with a prescription for fluconazole tablets. She is to take 150 mg by mouth daily for 3 days. On the shelf in the pharmacy you find 100-mg tablets. The pharmacist asks the patient if she is willing to use the 100-mg tablets and she agrees.
   a. How many tablets will you dispense?
   b. How will the directions on the prescription read?

7. Mrs. Berry is a frequent customer at Small's Pharmacy. Her 7-month-old, 16-pound son has a fever of 103°F. She asks you to double-check her dose calculation, based on the dose of ibuprofen the pharmacist recommended of 10 mg/kg with a maximum of four doses/day.

   a. How much ibuprofen should the baby receive per dose? *73 mg*

   b. Mrs. Berry chooses ibuprofen children's suspension, which contains 100 mg ibuprofen in 5 mL. What volume of ibuprofen will her son receive per dose in Part a? *OK convert lbs - kgs*

8. Convert the following weights to kilograms:

   a. 210 lb   b. 14 lb   c. 181 lb   d. 93 lb

9. Convert the following weights to pounds:

   a. 17.7 kg   b. 106 kg   c. 65 kg   d. 36 kg

10. Determine the volume of each dose of the following U100 insulin orders:

    a. Lantus insulin, 22 units daily at HS

    b. NPH U100 insulin, 45 units Q 12H

    c. Lispro insulin, 7 units before each meal

11. How many days will a 10-mL vial of insulin last, when used correctly, for each of the orders above?

12. Find the body surface area (BSA) for the heights and weights listed. If using an Internet calculator, round to the nearest hundredth.

    a. 5'9" and 168 lb

    b. 6'3" and 265 lb

    c. 5'2" and 131 kg

    d. 4'2" and 68 lb

    e. 96 cm and 16 kg

13. You need to prepare a syringe of heparin containing 22,500 units. The vial of heparin contains 10,000 units per mL. What volume of heparin will you draw up?

14. If a patient buys a 16-ounce bottle of Pepto-Bismol and plans on taking two tablespoonfuls twice a day while he is traveling in Central America, how long will the bottle last him?

15. An oncologist has ordered vinblastine 4 mg/m² to be given every week by slow IV push. The patient weighs 115 pounds and is 62 inches tall. What is the weekly dose (mg) of vinblastine? Patient's BSA = 1.5 m².

16. Annie Tyler is going to college and wants to take enough of her albuterol inhaler to last until she comes home at Thanksgiving, about 16 weeks. On average, she uses 2 puffs, 4 times each week. One canister provides around 200 inhalations. How many canisters will she need?

17. There is a levothyroxine injection shortage and the hospital has four postoperative patients that need this medication. The pharmacy will draw up a syringe for the patients, but a new single-dose vial must be used each day. The doses are as follows: 125 mcg, 0.175 mg, 100 mcg, and 0.075 mg each day. Each vial contains 0.5 mg levothyroxine.

    a. What is the total amount of levothyroxine used each day?

    b. The hospital has 8 vials left. How long will they last?

UNIT 4

18. A pharmacy technician is making penicillin G 4-million unit piggyback bags. She has two full 20-mL vials of penicillin G that have been reconstituted to 500,000 units per mL. How many 4-million unit piggyback bags can she make? *5 bags*

19. A prescriber orders acetaminophen 10-grain suppository for a bedridden hospice patient, whose husband comes in to pick up the medication. The pharmacy carries acetaminophen suppositories in 120-mg, 325-mg, and 650-mg strengths. Which strength should he purchase?

20. Your mother has been recently diagnosed with diabetes and she needs help calculating her insulin dose. She is to take Humalog® 5 units before each meal and she is to add additional units if her blood sugar is elevated. Her goal blood sugar is 130. She is to add 1 unit for every 40 points over the goal. She is due to eat lunch and her blood sugar is 250. What dose of Humalog® should she inject?

For problems 21–24, refer to the case below:

A physician has ordered Trileptal® suspension 300 mg/5 mL for a boy with a seizure disorder. The child is to receive 10 mg/kg/day initially, in two divided doses, with the dose to be increased gradually over time. The child weighs 44 pounds.

21. What is the child's weight in kg, and how much Trileptal® will he receive initially, per day, and per dose?

22. The physician orders that the boy's dose of Trileptal® be increased on the third day of treatment by 5 mg/kg/day divided in two doses. What is the new daily dose in mg/kg/day and how many mg of Trileptal® does he receive per dose? *15 mg   20 × 15 = 300/2 50 150mg per dose*

23. Eventually the child's dose is increased until he is receiving Trileptal® suspension 600 mg BID. What volume will his mother measure to deliver a 600-mg dose of the medication? *10 ml*

24. When the mother comes to the pharmacy to refill the Trileptal®, the new prescription reads as follows:

> Rx: Trileptal suspension 300 mg/5 mL, 1-month supply
> Sig: 600 mg BID = 1200mg

1200 × 30 = 36000 mg

What volume of the drug should the pharmacy supply to last 1 month?

25. Tracy Tan is a 20-month-old girl with a serious bacterial infection. Her physician orders ceftriaxone 50 mg/kg/day, in two divided doses, to be started immediately. Tracy weighs 21.5 pounds.

   a. What is Tracy's weight in kg? *9.8 kg*

   b. How many mg of ceftriaxone will Tracy receive per day and per dose? Round the daily dose to the nearest 100 mg.

CHAPTER 11

Percent Strengths and Dilutions

LEARNING OBJECTIVES

1. Define the terms *percent strength, weight-in-weight, weight-in-volume,* and *volume-in-volume.*
2. Convert a ratio, a fraction, and a decimal fraction to a percent.
3. Explain how to decide if a percent strength is a w/w, w/v, or v/v strength.
4. Find the percent strength of a product when two volumes of given strengths of the same ingredient are combined.
5. Use alligation appropriately in an alligation problem, and solve.

UNIT 4

Introduction

In Chapter 9 you were introduced to the concept of ratios and ratio strengths. The topic of strengths and concentrations continues here with more in-depth discussion of how these concepts are applied in pharmacy practice. You will continue to use ratio and proportion equations and other problem-solving strategies to solve problems that are centered on percents. A thorough understanding of percentage calculations, concentrations, and dilutions prepares pharmacy technician students for the rigorous requirements for accuracy when compounding drug preparations, in every pharmacy setting.

Percent Strengths

Outside of pharmacy practice, percentage calculations are employed to determine everything from sale discounts to grades in a class. Most high school graduates have an understanding of the concept of percent. As a quick review, remember that the word percent means "per 100." In other words, a percent is a ratio expressed in relationship to 100. Percents may be written as ratios, fractions or as decimal fractions. To convert a fraction to a percent, simply divide the numerator by the denominator, move the decimal two places to the right, and add a percent sign (%).

EXAMPLE

Write the fraction 4/5 as a decimal fraction and then convert it to a percent.

SOLUTION ···

$$5\overline{)4.0} \begin{array}{c} 0.8 \end{array}$$

$$0.80. = 80\%$$

Write 18% as a ratio strength, fraction, or decimal fraction.

SOLUTION ···

18:100, 18/100, and 0.18

Percent strength labeling occurs quite commonly on food and beverage packaging. If you read labels, you may have noticed products in your refrigerator or on your kitchen shelves that include percent strength labeling. A number of product labels, including vinegar (percent acidity) good quality chocolate (percent of cocoa in the final product), flavor extracts, like vanilla or almond extract (percent strength), and alcoholic beverages (percent alcohol) include concentration information as a percent. In pharmacy, we use the same basic concept. Percent still means parts per 100 parts, but technicians must be aware of the specific units of measure assigned to the parts.

First, take a moment to make certain you understand the concepts of strength and concentration. When discussing medication, **strength** refers to the labeled potency of a tablet or capsule, or other drug product. The terms *strength* or *concentration* may describe the amount of a specific compound in a defined weight or volume of a mixture. A **percent strength** is the concentration of an active ingredient or drug, represented as a percent, in a formulation or mixture.

Percent weight-in-volume

Drugs can be mixed in many different substances to produce a variety of finished medication formulations. The simplest kind of mixture is a solution, where a weighed soluble component is dissolved in a volume of fluid to produce the desired concentration of drug in the final product. There are specific terms used to describe the different components of a solution. The dissolved component is called the **solute**, the fluid in which it is dissolved is called the **solvent**, and the final formulation is called a **solution**. To make a solution, the solute is weighed on an accurate balance. The weighed solute is placed in a volumetric container, and fluid is added to make the desired volume. The percent strength of a solution made this way is referred to as percent weight-in-volume (w/v) because the solute is weighed and the final product is a liquid measured by volume. A percent strength (w/v) in pharmacy is always written as grams of solute per 100 mL solution, or grams/100 mL, unless otherwise indicated.

You decide to make simple syrup for an upcoming party, so your guests can mix it in their iced tea. The recipe asks you to measure 100 grams of granulated sugar, and add 100 mL of water. You dissolve the sugar by heating it just until it boils then cool it to room temperature and store it in the refrigerator. The recipe makes 150 mL of syrup. What percent strength is the finished syrup?

SOLUTION ···

The weight of the solute (the sugar) in this example is 100 g and the final volume of the solution is 150 mL, so the concentration is 100 g sugar/150 mL solution. This is the known ratio or concentration. In order to write this con-

Strength—Labeled potency of a tablet, capsule, or other drug product.

Percent Strength—The concentration of an active ingredient or drug, represented as a percent, in a formulation or mixture.

Solute—The substance dissolved in a solution.

Solvent—The liquid in which a solute is dissolved to form a solution.

Solution—A liquid preparation of one or more substances dissolved in a solvent.

centration as a percent strength, you need to calculate the amount of sugar in 100 mL of the solution.

$$\frac{100 \text{ g sugar}}{150 \text{ mL solution}} = \frac{x}{100 \text{ mL solution}}$$

$$\frac{x \,(\cancel{150 \text{ mL}})}{\cancel{150 \text{ mL}}} = \frac{(100 \text{ g}) (100 \,\cancel{\text{mL}})}{150 \,\cancel{\text{mL}}}$$

$$x = \frac{(100 \text{ g}) (100)}{150} = 66.7 \text{ g}$$

Therefore, our simple syrup concentration is 66.7g sugar/100 mL solution or 66.7%.

You can also solve this problem by simply dividing the numerator (100 g sugar) by the denominator (150 mL). The answer will be the decimal fraction 0.667. To convert to a percent, simply move the decimal two places to the right and add a percent sign.

Percent weight-in-volume calculations are used whenever a dry ingredient is dissolved in a liquid and are very common in pharmacy practice. Other examples would include calculations of percent strength of saline solutions, potassium chloride solutions, amino acid solutions, and many other drug solutions. Where drug products are concerned, you will usually be able to identify a weight-in-volume strength by reading the product label, which will clearly indicate a number of grams per volume, as seen in Figure 11-1.

Figure 11-1. The label shown indicates the product is a weight-in-volume solution with a labetalol concentration of 20 mg/4 mL (5 mg/mL).

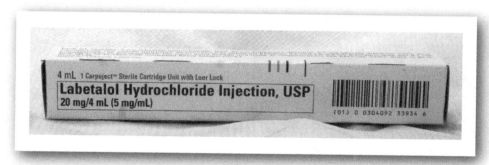

Source: Printed with permission from Hospira, Inc.

EXAMPLE

A lactulose solution contains 10 g lactulose in 15 mL. What is the percent strength of this product?

SOLUTION ···

$$\frac{10 \text{ g}}{15 \text{ mL}} = \frac{x}{100 \text{ mL}}$$

$$15 \text{ mL} \,(x) = (10 \text{ g})(100 \text{ mL})$$

$$x = \frac{10 \text{ g} \,(100 \text{ mL})}{15 \text{ mL}} = 66.7 \text{ g}$$

Therefore the w/v percent strength is 66.7 g/100 mL or 66.7%.

Percent weight-in-weight

Not every product used in a pharmacy is measured by volume. Creams, ointments, powders, and other solid or semisolid products are weighed. To calculate percent strength of a product measured by weight, compare the weight of the active ingredient to the total weight of the finished product. This kind of percent is referred to as weight-in-weight (w/w). Theoretically, any units may be used in the numerator as long as they are compared to 100 of the same units in the denominator. However, it is important for technician students to get comfortable with the metric system, so we will always compare grams of the ingredient to 100 grams when discussing w/w problems.

EXAMPLE

A canister of Desenex® powder is labeled as miconazole 2% powder. If the total weight of the powder is 85 grams, how many grams of miconazole does it contain?

SOLUTION ··

$$\frac{2 \text{ grams}}{100 \text{ grams}} = \frac{x}{85 \text{ grams}}$$

$$100 \text{ g } (x) = 2 \text{ g } (85 \text{ g})$$

$$x = 1.7 \text{ g}$$

Pharmacy technicians may be asked to compound a product that is not commercially available, from a formula, in order to meet the needs of a patient. Production of a medication in an appropriate quantity and dosage form using pharmaceutical ingredients on demand is called **extemporaneous compounding**. Take a look at the example that follows.

Extemporaneous Compounding—The production of a medication that is not commercially available, in an appropriate dosage form and quantity, from pharmaceutical ingredients.

EXAMPLE

Dr. Gutman calls in the following prescription to Scripts-R-Us compounding pharmacy.

> Rx: Hydrocortisone suppositories
> Hydrocortisone   100 mg
> Karaya gum   500 mg
> Base   1.4 g
> Disp: #12

What is the percent strength of hydrocortisone in each suppository?

SOLUTION ··

To calculate the percent of hydrocortisone in each suppository, first find the combined weight of all the ingredients. In order to add the weights listed, we will need to convert weights expressed in milligrams to grams.

Hydrocortisone 100 mg = 0.1 g
Karaya gum 500 mg =   0.5 g
Base   1.4 g
Total weight per suppository =   2 g

The known ratio 0.1 g hydrocortisone/2 g suppository represents the strength of hydrocortisone. Use a ratio and proportion equation to solve (or simply divide and convert to a percent by moving the decimal two places to the right).

$$\frac{0.1\ g}{2\ g} = \frac{x}{100\ g}$$

$$x\ (2g) = 0.1g\ (100\ g)$$

$$x = 5\ g$$

Therefore, the weight-in-weight strength per suppository is 5 g/100 g or 5% hydrocortisone.

Percent volume-in-volume

Percent volume-in-volume (v/v) problems are solved in much the same way as other percent concentration problems, except that the ingredients are all measured by volume. This type of problem is less common than the other two (w/v and w/w) problem types. As with weight-in-weight problems, units in the numerator and denominator must be the same; in v/v problems use of milliliters per 100 mL is the standard.

EXAMPLE

The local dentist, Dr. Doug Drilling, has a mouthwash formula that contains 0.25% spearmint oil for flavoring. The pharmacist wants you to make a pint of the mouthwash. How much spearmint oil will you need?

SOLUTION ···

The concentration of spearmint oil is 0.25% or 0.25 mL per 100 mL of mouthwash. A pint (16 oz) is approximately 480 mL. Use a ratio and proportion equation to solve.

$$\frac{0.25\ mL}{100\ mL} = \frac{x}{480\ mL}$$

$$x\ (100\ mL) = 0.25\ mL\ (480\ mL)$$

$$x = 1.2\ mL$$

You can also use dimensional analysis to solve this equation:

$$\frac{0.25\ mL}{100\ mL} \times \frac{480\ mL}{pint} = 0.0025\ (480\ mL)/pint =$$

1.2 mL spearmint oil/pint mouthwash

Milligrams percent and parts per million

Although not routinely used in medication dosing, technician students should be aware of another type of percent used by clinical laboratories to measure levels of drugs, glucose, electrolytes and other chemicals in the blood. Clinical laboratory results are often reported as mg%, or mg/dL meaning milligrams per 100 mL (also known as a deciliter, dL). This is a type of weight per volume concentration, but because the measured amount is so small, the weighed constituent is measured in mg instead of g.

The concentration of minute quantities in solution are expressed as parts per million (ppm). Parts per million refers to one gram per million grams or 1 gram per million milliliters of solution. This way of expressing a concentration is most frequently seen in discussions of additives, contaminants, or pollutants in water supplies or air.

Concentrated Solutions and Dilutions

In pharmacy, drugs, fluids, or electrolytes are sometimes supplied as concentrated solutions that must be diluted before they are administered to patients. Concentrated solutions are referred to as **stock solutions** or **concentrates**, and contain a higher quantity of active ingredient, or solute, per volume than is normal for administration to a patient. You may already be familiar with this concept if you have ever purchased a concentrate used around your home, such as plant fertilizer, cleaning agents, or even juice.

Concentrates are used because they take up less room to store and they allow flexibility. A variety of strengths of a product can be made from a concentrated solution. One word of caution: drug concentrates, by definition, must be diluted before administration to patients.

There are also times when a drug that is not a concentrate needs to be diluted. This occurs quite commonly in pediatric practices where doses are small and must be diluted in order to be measured accurately. So, it is very important for a technician to distinguish between pharmaceuticals that are not for use without dilution, and drug products that may require dilution in some situations but not in others. Concentrated electrolyte solutions (such as potassium chloride, KCl) are considered high-risk drugs, because use without dilution can be catastrophic to the patient. High-risk concentrates are most often found in hospitals or in pharmacies where sterile compounding is preformed. These concentrated solutions must never be delivered undiluted to nursing units or patients. Be sure to read labels so you know the difference (see Figure 11-2).

Figure 11-2. Labels on concentrated products, such as nitroprusside and potassium chloride shown, indicate "must be diluted before use" or "not for direct injection." These items must never be delivered to patients or patient care areas as is.

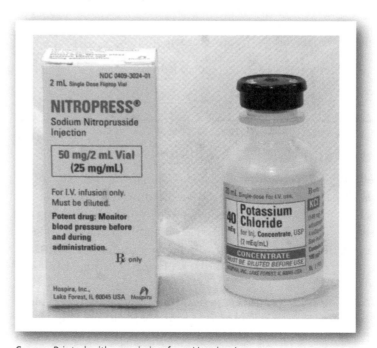

Source: Printed with permission from Hospira, Inc.

Stock Solutions—Solutions that contain a higher quantity of active ingredient, or solute, per volume than is normal for administration to a patient.

Concentrate—An increased strength of a pharmaceutical preparation used in compounding.

> ▶ *TECH NOTE!*
>
> **Concentrated solutions must never be delivered "as is" to patients or nursing units.**

Dilution means reduction of the concentration of a solute, or active ingredient, by addition of a diluent, which can be either a solvent or other inactive ingredient. In pharmacy practice, you may be asked to make sterile or non-sterile dilutions. Although dilution of a solution or other liquid is most common, a cream or ointment could also be diluted to make a lower concentration product. The key to working dilution problems is this: the amount of drug in a measured volume of concentrate is the same amount of drug that is in the diluted product. All that is needed is to determine the new concentration. Look at the following example.

Dilution—The process of making a pharmaceutical preparation less concentrated.

EXAMPLE

Povidone iodine 10% is to be diluted for a vaginal douche. The directions are to add 15 mL of 10% povidone iodine to 985 mL of water for irrigation. What is the percent concentration of povidone iodine in the diluted product?

SOLUTION ···

First, using the ratio and proportion method, determine the amount of pure povidone iodine in 15 mL of 10% povidone iodine solution.

$$\frac{10\ g}{100\ mL} = \frac{x}{15\ mL}$$

$$100\ mL\ (x) = 15\ mL\ (10\ g)$$

$$x = \frac{15\ mL\ (10\ g)}{100\ mL}$$

$$x = 1.5\ g\ povidone\ iodine\ in\ 15\ mL\ 10\%\ solution$$

Now we know the amount of povidone iodine in the final solution, 1.5 g. We also know the total volume of the final solution. We added 985 mL of water to our initial volume of 15 mL.

$$15\ mL + 985\ mL = 1000\ mL$$

The last step in the problem is to determine the new concentration as a percent, again using the ratio and proportion method.

$$\frac{1.5\ g}{1000\ mL} = \frac{x}{100\ mL}$$

$$x\ (1000\ mL) = 1.5\ g\ (100\ mL)$$

$$x = \frac{1.5\ g\ (100\ mL)}{1000\ mL}$$

$$x = 0.15\ g$$

So, the diluted solution is 0.15 g povidone iodine per 100 mL or 0.15% povidone iodine solution.

The previous example demonstrated how to determine the final concentration of a solution when the initial amount of drug added was known. More often the final concentration is given and the technician will need to determine what volume of concentrate to add to achieve the end product. In this type of problem, you will determine the amount of drug in the final product first, and work backwards to determine the volume of concentrate that contains that needed amount.

> ### ▶ TECH NOTE!
>
> *For safety reasons, always estimate before you calculate and double-check your answers.*

EXAMPLE

The children's hospital where you work uses 3% (hypertonic) sodium chloride for inhalation via nebulizer for infants with respiratory viral infections. The pharmacy makes 100 mL quantities using sterile water and sterile 23.4% NaCl (sodium chloride). What volume of the concentrated sodium chloride do you need to make 100 mL of the 3% solution? How much sterile water will you use? Estimate first!

SOLUTION ··

Remember, 23.4% means 23.4 grams in 100 mL, and 3% means 3 g in 100 mL. To estimate, think in rounded numbers. If you round 23.4 g up to 30 grams, you can see that 100 mL of the concentrated NaCl is about 10 times what you need. Therefore, when you calculate the volume of concentrate you need to make the dilution, it should be around 10 mL. That means you will need about 90 mL of sterile water to make 100 mL of the diluted solution.

Now, look at the calculation. You need 3 g of sodium chloride, and you know there are 23.4 grams NaCl in every 100 mL of the concentrate. Use the ratio and proportion method to calculate the volume of concentrate needed to provide 3 g NaCl.

$$\frac{23.4\ g}{100\ mL} = \frac{3\ g}{x}$$

$$x\ (23.4\ g) = 100\ mL\ (3\ g)$$

$$x = \frac{100\ mL\ (3\ g)}{23.4\ g}$$

$$x = 12.8\ mL\ concentrated\ NaCl$$

Because we estimated first, we know that an answer of 12.8 mL is within reason. Next subtract 12.8 mL from the final volume of 100 mL to determine the amount of sterile water that, when added, will make 100 mL of 3% NaCl.

100 mL 3% NaCl volume – 12.8 mL NaCl concentrate = 87.2 mL sterile water

Sometimes dilutions used in pharmacy are not quite this straight forward. There are usually multiple ingredients that add volume to the final product when compounding solutions for intravenous use. In a case where multiple ingredients are combined, the total volume of all ingredients needs to be included in the calculations.

EXAMPLE

You are to make a 1000 mL total parenteral nutrition solution (TPN, used for intravenous feeding) with a final concentration of 20% dextrose. You have dextrose 70% and sterile water on hand. The TPN will also contain 500 mL amino acid solution, 7.5 mL vitamins and trace metals and 28.5 mL electrolytes. How much 70% dextrose do you need to make the TPN? How much sterile water will you need to complete the product?

SOLUTION ··

You know that the final volume of the TPN is to be 1000 mL. First, calculate the volume of 70% dextrose needed to make one liter of 20% dextrose. Remember, 20% means 20 g/100 mL. Using dimensional analysis we see that:

$$20 \text{ g}/100 \text{ mL} \times 1000 \text{ mL/L} = 200 \text{ g/L of dextrose in a 20% solution}$$

You can also use ratio and proportion to complete this step. So, what volume of 70% dextrose will provide 200 g? Remember to estimate first!

$$\frac{70 \text{ g}}{100 \text{ mL}} = \frac{200 \text{ g}}{x}$$

$$x \,(70\text{g}) = 200 \text{ g } (100 \text{ mL})$$

$$x = \frac{200 \text{ g } (100 \text{ mL})}{70 \text{ g}}$$

$$x = 285.7 \text{ mL}$$

Unless the pharmacy uses an automated compounding machine, this volume would be rounded to 285 mL. It is not possible to measure 285.7 mL accurately in an IV bag. This answer tells us that 285 mL of 70% dextrose contains 200 g dextrose, or enough dextrose to make one liter of 20% dextrose solution. Now, add the volume of the other ingredients:

$$500 \text{ mL amino acid soln} + 7.5 \text{ mL vits/trace metals} + 28.5 \text{ mL electrolytes} = 536 \text{ mL total}$$

Add the total volume of the solutions to the volume of 70% dextrose and subtract from 1000 mL determine how much sterile water needs to be added to make one liter of final product.

$$285 \text{ mL 20% dextrose} + 536 \text{ mL other ingredients} = 821 \text{ mL}$$
$$1000 \text{ mL} - 821 \text{ mL} = 179 \text{ mL sterile water}$$

Alligation medial

Alligation is a process used to solve compounding problems where a new strength is made from two or more strengths of one product. **Alligation medial** is the process used to find the strength of a product when known amounts of a given concentration are combined. In this process, the amount of drug in the ingredients is determined, and the measured volume or weight of the ingredients is totaled. These sums are then written as a ratio and the new percent strength is calculated.

Alligation—A practical method used to solve compounding problems where a new strength is made from two different strengths of the same product.

Alligation Medial—The process used to find the strength of a product when known amounts of a given concentration are combined. In this process, the amount of drug in the ingredients is determined, and the measured volume or weight of the ingredients is totaled. These sums are then written as a ratio and the new percent strength is calculated.

EXAMPLE

While working at the pharmacy, you receive the following prescription:

> Sita Rash, M.D.
> 149 Hive Lane,
> Weldon, CA
>
> For: Mona Groening   Date: 4/21/12
> Address: 4212 N. Main
>
> Rx: Triamcinolone 0.1% ointment
>   Triamcinolone 0.025% ointment
>   aa qs 60 g
>
> Refill: 0 _x_ 1___ 2___   _Sita Rash_   M.D.

The label will need to include the final strength of triamcinolone ointment. What strength is the final product?

SOLUTION ··

The abbreviations aa qs mean "of each to make." Therefore, the prescription calls for equal parts of each ingredient (30 g) to make a final weight of 60 g. First, calculate how much triamcinolone is in 30 grams of 0.1% and 30 gram of 0.025% triamcinolone ointment. Below, you can see how either the ratio and proportion method or dimensional analysis may be used to determine the weight of triamcinolone in each ingredient.

Ratio and proportion method for the 0.1% product:

$$\frac{0.1\ g}{100\ g} = \frac{x}{30\ g}$$

$$x\ (100\ g) = 0.1\ g\ (30\ g)$$
$$x = 0.03\ g\ \text{triamcinolone in 30 g of 0.1% ointment}$$

Dimensional analysis method for the 0.025% product:

$$0.025\ g/100\ g \times 30\ g = 0.0075\ g\ \text{triamcinolone in 30 g of 0.025% ointment}$$

To calculate the new strength of the triamcinolone ointment, add the weight of triamcinolone in the ingredients, and add the weight of the combined ingredients to create a new ratio:

$$\frac{0.03\ g + 0.0075\ g}{30\ g + 30\ g} = \frac{0.0375\ g}{60\ g}$$

$$\frac{0.0375\ g}{60\ g} = \frac{x}{100\ g}$$

$$x\ (60\ g) = 0.0375\ g\ (100\ g)$$

$$x = 0.0625\ g\ \text{per 100 g; therefore, the new strength is 0.0625%}$$

Table 11-1 describes this method as a formula you can use to calculate new percent strengths from a combination of different strengths of the same product. Notice that you can use the same formula for calculating weight-in-weight, weight-in-volume or volume-in-volume preparations, as long as the ingredients are just different strengths of the same product. Take a look at one more example of alligation medial.

Table 11-1. Method for Calculating the New Percent Strength as a Formula When Different Strengths of the Same Product Are Added Together in Known Measures

$$\frac{A + B + C}{M_a + M_b + M_c} = \frac{X}{100}$$

1. A, B and C are the weight or volume of the *active ingredient* in each strength of the product used.

2. M_a, M_b, and M_c are the *measured total weights or volumes* of each product used.

3. Set the new ratio up as a ratio and proportion equation, where X is the new percent strength.

EXAMPLE

Patsy is graduating from her pharmacy technician program and decides to make punch for her party that contains a liter of grapefruit juice, two liters of lemon-lime soda, 473 mL of vodka (40% alcohol) and 750 mL of champagne (12% alcohol). What is the alcohol (in this case, the active ingredient) content of the punch?

SOLUTION ···

Use the formula illustrated in Table 11-1 for practice. Notice the juice and soda have no alcohol, but their volume must be added in the denominator. Calculate the volume of pure alcohol in the vodka and champagne before you look at the answer below to test your understanding of the process.

$$\frac{0 \text{ mL} + 0 \text{ mL} + 189.2 \text{ mL (vodka)} + 90 \text{ mL (champagne)}}{1000 \text{ mL} + 2000 \text{ mL} + 473 \text{ mL} + 750 \text{ mL}} = \frac{279.2 \text{ mL}}{4223 \text{ mL}} = 6.6\% \text{ alcohol punch}$$

Alligation alternate

Alligation alternate is an approach used to solve a different type of strength calculation problem. The alligation medial method described above can be used to determine the new strength of any combination of strengths as long as you know the amount of each. It can be used to create a specific strength from combining a known concentration and a diluent of 0% concentration, as well. The alligation alternate method is used to calculate how much of each of two strength products should be combined to create a new product of intermediate specified strength.

To further examine the difference in the two methods, consider how the problem above would be solved if Dr. Rash wanted the pharmacy to make 0.05% triamcinolone cream instead of the 0.0625%. If the technician had a base cream with no triamcinolone and the 0.1% triamcinolone the calculation could be made using the alligation medial process. If, however, only the 0.1% triamcinolone and 0.025% triamcinolone cream were available, the technician might be able to get close to the amounts to use through trial and error with the alligation medial process, but getting to the exact concentration this way would be dependent upon a

UNIT

4

Alligation Alternate—
Alligation alternate is an approach used to solve a different type of strength calculation problem. The alligation alternate method is used to calculate how much of each of two strength products should be combined to create a new product of intermediate specified strength.

lucky guess. Alligation alternate is a way to determine the exact amount needed of two ingredients to get the desired concentration in the final product.

Solving an alligation alternate problem is a two-step process. The first step uses an alligation grid (Figure 11-3) and provides you with the ratio of the higher strength ingredient to the lower strength ingredient in terms of "parts" of each. The parts have no assigned units of measure. The second step involves changing that ratio of parts into actual measurements. The new triamcinolone cream problem will be used to demonstrate this process.

Figure 11-3. This example of an alligation grid shows how to determine the relative parts of each product used to make a new desired strength.

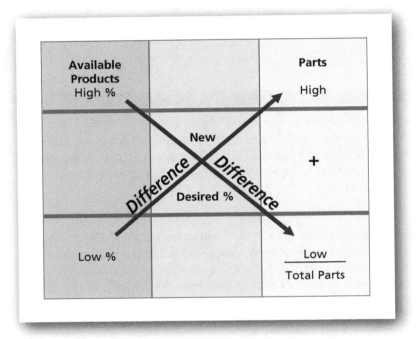

EXAMPLE

Use alligation alternate to figure out how to combine triamcinolone 0.1% ointment with triamcinolone 0.025% ointment to make 60 g of triamcinolone 0.05% ointment.

SOLUTION ···

Here is the alligation alternate method, step-by-step.

Step 1. Create an alligation grid (think tic-tac-toe).

Step 2. The left side of the grid is where you will keep track of the products you are mixing. In the upper left hand corner of the grid write the higher concentration strength (0.1%). Write the lower concentration in the lower left corner (0.025%).

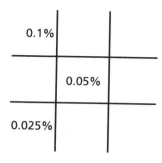

Step 3. Write the desired concentration (new product) in the center of the grid (0.05%).

Step 4. Find the difference of the lower concentration and desired concentration and write it in the upper right corner. This number tells you how many parts you will use of the higher concentration product (0.025). Find the difference of the higher concentration and desired concentration and write it in the lower right hand corner. This number tells you how many parts you will use of the lower concentration product (0.05).

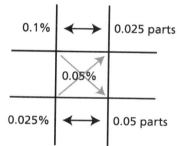

total parts: 0.075

Step 5. Add the parts of the low and high concentration components (0.025 + 0.05 = 0.075). Set up a ratio of high concentration parts to total parts and set it equal to a ratio with x in the numerator and 60 g in the denominator, the total amount of ointment you are making.

$$\frac{0.025 \text{ parts}}{0.075 \text{ parts}} = \frac{x}{60 \text{ g}}$$

$$x(0.075) = (0.025)60 \text{ g}$$

$$x = \frac{(0.025)\ 60 \text{ g}}{0.075} = 20 \text{ g of } 0.1\% \text{ triamcinolone ointment}$$

Step 6. Set up a ratio of low concentration parts to total parts and proceed as in Step 5.

$$\frac{0.05 \text{ parts}}{0.075 \text{ parts}} = \frac{x}{60 \text{ g}}$$

$$x(0.075) = (0.05)\ 60 \text{ g}$$

$$x = \frac{(0.05)\ 60 \text{ g}}{0.075} = 40 \text{ g of } 0.025\% \text{ triamcinolone ointment}$$

Step 7. Now, check your calculations to verify that the sum of the calculated parts adds up to the desired quantity of 0.05% triamcinolone ointment you wish to make.

20 g (of 0.1%) + 40 g (of 0.025%) = 60 grams ointment

Although this may seem like a complicated solution to an unlikely request, these problems do arise in pharmacy practice. Perhaps a more relevant issue for pharmacy technician students is the possibility that alligation alternate problems may appear on the national pharmacy certification exam, so it is important to master this type of problem. With that in mind, look at another example. This example comes from situations that arise in hospital pharmacy practice.

EXAMPLE

A physician orders a total parenteral nutrition (TPN) solution with dextrose 17.5%. The pharmacist explains that you will need 500 mL of 35% dextrose to make the correct concentration of dextrose in the final product. Your job is to make 500 mL of 35% dextrose from the dextrose 50% and dextrose 20% on the shelf. Use the alligation alternate method to decide how much of each product to use.

SOLUTION

First, fill out the alligation grid.

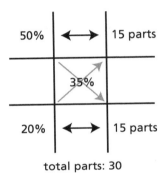

total parts: 30

In this particular problem, you should immediately notice that the solution requires equal parts of each component. Clearly, we already have an answer: to make 500 mL of 35% dextrose, add 250 mL each of 50% and 20% dextrose. But for the sake of practice, let's go through the math.

$$\frac{15 \text{ parts}}{30 \text{ parts}} = \frac{x}{500 \text{ mL}}$$

$$x \,(30 \text{ parts}) = 15 \text{ parts} \,(500 \text{ mL})$$

$$x = \frac{15 \text{ parts} \,(500 \text{ mL})}{30 \text{ parts}} = 250 \text{ mL}$$

In summary, you can use the alligation methods described here to compound a product in a strength that is not readily available. As long as you have a product strength higher than the needed strength, one of the problem solving methods described in this chapter will work. If you are mixing two measured amounts of two known strengths and wish to find the new strength, use alligation medial. To make a new product concentration in a specified amount using two different strengths, use alligation alternate to determine how much of each product to mix.

Practice Problems

1. Write the following as percents:

 a. 0.15   b. 22/100   c. 0.63   d. ¾   e. 1.1   f. 17/24

2. Write the following as percents:

 a. 0.75   b. 33/100   c. 0.81   d. 5/8   e. 1.2   f. 3/25

3. From the labels shown, decide whether percentage strengths would be w/w or w/v.

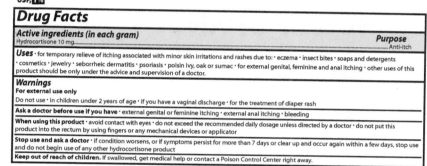

a.

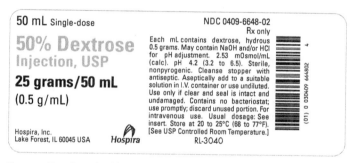

b. *Source:* Reprinted with permission of Hospira, Inc.

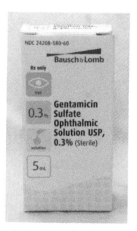

c. *Source:* Reprinted with permission of Bausch & Lomb, Inc.

4. Write the following percents as ratios, including appropriate units:
   a. 5% (w/v)   b. 24% (w/w)   c. 0.1% (v/v)

5. Write the following percents as ratios, including appropriate units:
   a. 0.9% (w/v)   b. 0.75% (v/v)   c. 10% (w/w)

6. You dispense 480 mL of the KCl 10% liquid shown here. How many grams are in this volume of KCl oral solution?

POTASSIUM CHLORIDE ORAL SOLUTION, USP 10% SF ORANGE

Each 15 mL (tablespoonful) contains: 20 mEq of potassium chloride (provided by potassium chloride 1.5 g), in a palatable, orange flavored, sugar free vehicle, alcohol 4.0%.
Inactive ingredients" Citric acid, FD&C Yellow #6, flavor, methylparaben, propylene glycol, propylparaben, purified water, saccharin sodium, sorbitol.
DOSAGE AND ADMINISTRATION: See package insert for complete dosage recommendations.
MUST BE DILUTED.
DISPENSE in a tight, light-resistant container as defined in the USP/NF.
STORE at 20 to 25 C (68 to 77 F) (see USP Controlled Room Temperature).
AVOID FREEZING.

Rx only

NET: 1 PINT (473 mL)

7. How much pure ethanol is in 500 mL 70% (v/v) ethanol solution?

8. The pure vanilla extract on grandma's shelf contains 35% ethyl alcohol. She has an 8-fl oz bottle.
   a. How much alcohol is in 100 mL of vanilla extract?
   b. How much alcohol is contained in the full 8-fl oz bottle?

9. You are asked to make 240 mL of 3% hydrogen peroxide from the available 6% hydrogen peroxide solution and sterile water for irrigation. How much of each ingredient is needed to make the preparation? (Note: 3% hydrogen peroxide is half as strong as 6%.)

10. When you go in for a physical examination you learn that your blood glucose is normal at 77 mg/dL.
    a. What is your blood sugar level in mg%?
    b. What is your blood sugar level expressed as g/100 mL (%w/v)?

11. Dexamethasone for injection is available as 4 mg/mL and 10 mg/mL. What are the percent strengths of each product?

12. Timolol ophthalmic drops are available in 0.25% and 0.5% concentrations.
    a. How many milligrams of timolol are in a 10-mL bottle of 0.25% solution?
    b. How many milligrams of timolol are in a 15-mL bottle of 0.5% solution?

13. It is a hot summer day in Southern California where you are vacationing, and you hear on the radio that carbon monoxide levels are above the healthy range at 11 PPM. Express this concentration as a percent and as a ratio.

14. An injectable antibiotic is provided as 80 mg/2 mL. Write this ratio as a percent strength.

15. You are to compound one pound of 3% hydrocortisone cream from cream base and hydrocortisone powder.
    a. How much hydrocortisone is contained in one pound of the cream?
    b. How much of the cream base is needed for this product?
    c. Is this a w/w or w/v problem?

16. A patient is receiving an IV of 5% dextrose in water. The dextrose solution is infusing at a rate of 125 mL every hour.
    a. How many grams of dextrose will the patient receive in 1 hour?
    b. How many grams of dextrose will the patient receive in 1 day?

17. Bumetanide injection contains bumetanide 1 mg/mL. What is the percent strength?

18. A saline solution contains 2.25 grams sodium chloride in 250 mL. What is the percent strength of this solution?

19. Mometasone cream contains 45 mg mometasone in 45 grams of cream. What percent strength is the cream?

20. What is the percent strength of benzalkonium chloride if equal parts of 2% and 6% benzalkonium chloride are mixed together?

21. You are making a 1-liter intravenous solution with 250 mL of 50% dextrose and 750 mL of amino acids, electrolytes, and sterile water.
    a. What is the final concentration of dextrose in the 1-liter bag?
    b. Of the 750 mL added to the dextrose, 500 mL is 7% amino acids solution. What is the final concentration of amino acids in 1 liter?

22. In the hospital pharmacy where you work, the pharmacist receives an order for 500 mL dextrose 10%. Unfortunately, this particular IV solution was not ordered and the pharmacy is out, but you do have dextrose 5% and dextrose 20%. How much of each solution is needed to make 500 mL of dextrose 10%?

23. The local veterinarian would like 10 mL of phenobarbital for injection in a 7.5% solution. You have on hand 65 mg/mL and 130 mg/mL.
    a. What are the percent strengths of the 65 mg/mL and 130 mg/mL solutions for injection?
    b. How many mL of each strength phenobarbital for injection is needed to make 10 mL of 7.5% solution?

24. An antibiotic flush solution made by the hospital pharmacy contains vancomycin 25 mcg/mL and ciprofloxacin 2 mcg/mL. Write these concentrations as mg % strengths.

25. Normal saline solution contains 0.9% sodium chloride (NaCl). Other saline solutions are known as ½ normal saline and ¼ normal saline, because they are ½ and ¼ the concentration of normal saline.

   a. What is the percent strength of ½ normal saline?

   b. What is the percent strength of ¼ normal saline?

Formulas and Compounding

UNIT 4

LEARNING OBJECTIVES

1. Perform the calculations necessary to reduce or enlarge a compounding formula.
2. Knowing the sensitivity rating and expected % error, determine the minimum weighable quantity for a pharmacy balance.
3. Explain the use of aliquots for measuring small amounts of drugs.
4. Calculate either mass, volume, or density of a compound when given the other two.
5. Determine percent error when given a measured value and true value.

Introduction

Production of a medication that is not commercially available, in an appropriate dosage form and quantity, from pharmaceutical ingredients, is called extemporaneous compounding. Almost all pharmacies compound, or mix, products to meet the needs of patients to some extent, and some pharmacies specialize in extemporaneous compounding of products. All pharmacy technicians need to understand the basic math involved with compounding and quality control of the resulting products.

Understanding Compounding Formulas

The concept of compounding pharmacies and formulas might conjure up visions of chemists at lab tables with bubbling beakers and fuming flasks. A more accurate analogy of a compounding pharmacy is a very clean and automated kitchen, just as a formula could be compared to a recipe. As you will recall, the abbreviation *Rx* stands for the Latin "recipere."

In pharmacy, compounding formulas list all the necessary active and inactive ingredients, along with instructions for preparation, quality control, labeling and beyond-use dating. Frequently used formulas are kept on a master formula sheet or record and stored where they are easily accessible. Figure 12-1 is an example of a master formula record. As a reminder, Table 7-2 in Chapter 7 lists a number of Latin abbreviations that you may encounter when using a compounding formula.

Reducing and enlarging formulas

If you have ever prepared a dish from a recipe, you know that there are times when the recipe provides too much or not enough finished product to meet your needs. The same can be true of pharmacy compounding formulas. When that occurs, the formula must be reduced or enlarged. Look at the following example, which describes enlarging a lemonade recipe.

Figure 12-1. An example of a master formula record.

Compounding Laboratory
Pharmacy Technician Training Program

Name of Formulation: Wintergreen Sports Rub
Formula Amount: 100 g

Ingredients	Form	Recipe Amount
1. Methyl Salicylate	oil	30 g
2. Menthol	crystals	7.5 g
3. Lanolin	ointment	7.5 g
4. White petrolatum	ointment	55 g

Preparation:

1. Incorporate the lanolin into the white petrolatum.

2. Dissolve the menthol in the oil of wintergreen (methyl salicylate).

3. Incorporate the menthol/methyl salicylate into the white petrolatum.

4. Mix well.

5. Package and label.

    Special labeling: External use only

    Storage and stability: Store at controlled room temperature

    Beyond-use-date: 1 year

EXAMPLE

Your grandmother's lemonade recipe serves 6 and you are expecting 12 guests for lunch. How do you enlarge the recipe to serve everyone?

Lemonade

1 cup freshly squeezed lemon juice
¾ cup sugar
6 cups water

SOLUTION ···

You need to increase the amount of each ingredient equally so that the relationship of the ingredients to each other remains the same. Since you are serving 12 people, you must multiply each ingredient by 2, since 6 × 2 = 12, so you would double the recipe; 2 cups lemon juice, 1½ cups sugar, and 12 cups water.

EXAMPLE

Two guests cancelled for your luncheon. Now only ten people are coming and you decide to reduce the doubled lemonade recipe. Now the question is, how do you reduce your recipe?

SOLUTION ···

To find a factor to reduce or enlarge a recipe or a compounding formula, divide the needed amount by the amount the formula provides. Each ingredient is then multiplied by this factor. In the case of the lemonade we are referring to "servings," but the same rule applies to other units, as long as they are the same. Another way to think of this is what number multiplied by 12 servings gives you 10 servings?

$$(x)12 = 10$$
$$x = 10/12$$
$$x = 0.83 \text{ or rounded, } 0.8$$

So, multiply each ingredient in the enlarged formula by 0.8

2 c lemon juice (0.8) = 1.6 c lemon juice
1½ c sugar (0.8) = 1.6 c sugar
12 c water (0.8) = 9.6 c water

Clearly, this example is a little silly. Nobody would reduce their lemonade recipe in this way, because it would be too difficult to measure, and someone would drink the leftovers anyway. In pharmacy formulas, however, ingredients might be expensive and amounts dispensed must match the physician's prescription. Look at the sports rub formula in Figure 12-1 for the next example.

EXAMPLE

Dr. Joinz prescribed his Wintergreen Sports Rub for a member of the adult soccer league who hurt himself in the game. The prescription is for 150 g. What are the new amounts of each ingredient needed to make 150 g?

SOLUTION ···

The amount of sports rub needed is 150 g and the original formula makes 100 g. To determine the factor for increasing the formula, divide the amount needed by the amount the formula provides.

$$\frac{150 \text{ g}}{100 \text{ g}} = 1.5$$

Now, multiply each ingredient in the formula by 1.5. Check your calculations by verifying that the total weight of the new formula = 150 g.

Methyl salicylate 30 g (1.5) = 45 g
Menthol 7.5 g (1.5) = 11.25 g
Lanolin 7.5 g (1.5) = 11.25 g
White petrolatum 55 g (1.5) = 82.5 g

Total weight = 150 g

Using aliquots

An **aliquot** is a portion or part of a whole, where most often, the aliquot divides into the whole with no remainder. Aliquots are used in pharmacy when the desired amount of a drug is too small to safely or accurately measure using the available equipment. This kind of situation is quite common in pediatric settings and in compounding pharmacies.

To use the aliquot method, the minimum weighable quantity (MWQ) or least measurable quantity must be determined for the selected method of measurement. **Minimum weighable quantity** is the smallest amount that can be weighed with an acceptable error rate. When measuring liquid ingredients, the least measurable quantity is dependent upon the divisions (or graduations) on the syringe or other device used for liquid measurement. When weighing dry ingredients, this number depends on the sensitivity requirement of the balance you are using. The sensitivity requirement tells you the minimum amount that can be accurately weighed, and by inference, the increments that can be accurately measured. In other words, if your balance is sensitive to 10 mg, you could theoretically measure 20 mg, but not 21 mg, because the balance is not sensitive enough to register the difference between 20 and 21 mg. Table 12-1 shows the formula for calculating the minimum weighable quantity. Notice that the more precise you want the measurement to be, the larger the minimum weighable quantity becomes. In pharmacy, the standard acceptable error is 5%.

Table 12-1. Determining Minimum Weighable Quantity on a Pharmacy Balance

1. Determine the sensitivity rating for your balance.
2. Determine the permissible rate of error for your product (USP standard is 5% or less).
3. $$\frac{SR \times 100}{\% \text{ error}} = MWQ$$
4. Example: Your balance sensitivity rating is 10 mg and the permissible error is 5%.

$$\frac{10 \text{ mg} \times 100}{5} = 200 \text{ mg} = MWQ$$

Once the smallest measurable amount is determined, that amount is measured out and mixed with a measured amount of diluent. When the active ingredient is dispersed evenly within the diluent, an aliquot (or portion) that contains the desired amount of medication can be measured.

EXAMPLE

The neonatologist at Shoreside Children's Hospital orders furosemide 0.5 mg to be given IV × 1 for a premature newborn baby. Furosemide for injection comes from the manufacturer as 10 mg/1 mL. The pharmacist tells you to dilute 10 mg with normal saline so that the 0.5-mg dose is contained in 0.2 mL, the smallest measurable amount for a 1-mL syringe. How will you dilute this drug?

SOLUTION ···

The desired concentration is 0.5 mg/0.2 mL. You can use a ratio and proportion equation to answer the question, what volume will contain 10 mg if 0.2 mL contains 0.5 mg?

$$\frac{0.5 \text{ mg}}{0.2 \text{ mL}} = \frac{10 \text{ mg}}{x}$$

$$x \,(0.5 \text{ mg}) = 10 \text{ mg} \,(0.2 \text{ mL})$$

$$x = \frac{10 \text{ mg} \,(0.2 \text{ mL})}{0.5 \text{ mg}}$$

$$x = 4 \text{ mL}$$

The final volume of the diluted product will be 4 mL. The question is, how much normal saline is added to reach this concentration? At this point it is important to remember that the furosemide 10 mg already takes up 1 mL of the final volume. Subtract the volume of the furosemide (1 mL) from the final volume (4 mL) to determine the amount of saline to add.

4 mL final volume – 1 mL furosemide = 3 mL added diluent

Density and Specific Gravity

Although density and specific gravity problems are not common in pharmacy practice, an understanding of these concepts is useful in compounding. Density describes how much of a substance is packed into a particular space, and is unique for each substance. In more scientific terms, **density** is the mass of a substance per unit of volume it occupies, and is reported as g/mL.

$$\text{Density} = \frac{\text{mass}}{\text{volume}}$$

Density varies depending upon the temperature of the substance and the atmospheric pressure. The density of water, at standard temperature (4°C) and pressure (sea level), is 1 g/mL. A substance that is more dense than water will sink below it, and a substance that is less dense than water will float on top of it. Mineral oil is an example of a substance less dense than water, and glycerin is more dense.

Specific gravity is the relative density of a substance as compared to the density of water under the same conditions. If the density of any substance is divided by the density of water, all the units (grams and mL) will cancel, and the resulting answer is the specific gravity. If the specific gravity of a substance is greater than one, that substance is more dense than water, and if it is less than one it is less dense than water. Use the formula for density, above, to solve the following problems.

Density—The mass of a substance per unit of volume it occupies, reported as g/mL.

EXAMPLE

You are measuring out glycerin for a dry skin preparation. The formula calls for 32 grams of glycerin. While weighing the substance in a volumetric container, you notice that at room temperature, 32 grams of glycerin fills a volume of about 25.5 mL. What is the density of glycerin?

SOLUTION ··

$$\text{Density} = \frac{\text{mass}}{\text{volume}}$$

$$\text{Density of glycerin} = \frac{32 \text{ g}}{25.5 \text{ mL}} = 1.255 \text{ g/mL}$$

When the density of glycerin is divided by the density of water, the result is the specific gravity.

$$\frac{1.255 \text{ g/mL}}{1 \text{ g/mL}} = 1.255, \text{ the specific gravity of glycerin}$$

By working with this same formula, you can solve for an unknown mass or volume when density is known. Whether solving for mass or volume, by inputting the known information, you can solve for the necessary unknown.

EXAMPLE

You are weighing out 300 grams of 70% isopropyl alcohol but you are unsure of what size container to choose to hold this amount. The density of isopropyl alcohol at room temperature is 0.78 g/mL. Should you choose a 250-mL or 500-mL container?

SOLUTION ··

Plug the known values into the formula and solve for the unknown value, the volume of the alcohol.

$$0.78 \text{ g/mL} = \frac{300 \text{ g}}{x}$$

$$x \, (0.78 \text{ g/mL}) = 300 \text{ g}$$

$$x = \frac{300 \text{ g}}{0.78 \text{ g/mL}}$$

$$x = 384.6 \text{ mL}$$

You will need the 500-mL container to hold the alcohol.

Because density and specific gravity are unique for any given material, they are useful tools for measuring and analyzing a substance. For example, automated compounding machines may measure the mass of liquid ingredients then use density information to assure the correct volume. Pharmacy staff must input accurate density information into the computer software so that measurements are correct. This information is readily available in pharmacy references or on products themselves.

Determining Percent Error

Whenever something is measured in pharmacy, even with the best possible technique, there is a degree of variance inherent in the measurement. This variation from the true value occurs because of the limits of accuracy in measuring systems, user error, environmental variations, and even intentional variation, such as overfill, in a container. This variance is reported as percent error, and is calculated with the following formula.

$$\% \text{ error} = \frac{|\text{measured value - true value}|}{\text{true value}} \times 100$$

A measured value may be either above or below the true value, so percent errors are reported as a range around the true value. The vertical bars in the numerator indicate absolute value, meaning that the difference of the measured and true is always reported as a positive number.

EXAMPLE

An IV bag is labeled as 100 mL normal saline. Andy Ayrers, pharmacy technician student, is asked to measure the volume of the saline in a graduated cylinder and report the percent error. Andy empties the IV bag carefully and completely into a 250-mL graduate and squeezes out every last drop. Andy carefully reads the measurement at eye-level and finds that there is actually 105 mL normal saline in the bag. Now he needs to calculate percent error.

SOLUTION ···

Because Andy knows that manufacturers intentionally overfill IV bags, he will use his measurement as the more accurate "true value."

$$\% \text{ error} = \frac{|100 \text{ mL} - 105 \text{ mL}|}{105 \text{ mL}} \times 100$$

$$\% \text{ error} = \frac{5 \text{ mL}}{105 \text{ mL}} \times 100 = 4.8$$

Andy reports the percent error as 4.8%.

In the next chapter you will continue to learn how to solve problems related to compounding. Be sure to work the practice problems here so that you have a strong foundation to build upon.

Practice Problems

1. You work in a compounding pharmacy where the elderly gastroenterologist sends his patients for his special GI upset capsules. Each capsule contains hyoscyamine 0.1 mg, bismuth subsalicylate 500 mg, and famotidine 10 mg. The pharmacist asks you to make 150 capsules. How much of each ingredient will you need?

2. Mrs. Rose Easkin brings in a prescription for 6 ounces of coal tar ointment. The coal tar formula makes 8 ounces. By what factor will you multiply each ingredient to reduce the formula from 8 ounces to 6 ounces?

3. Advil® Cold and Sinus Caplets each contain ibuprofen 200 mg and pseudoephedrine 30 mg. How much of each ingredient will the manufacturer use to make a bottle of 60 caplets?

Answer Questions 4–6 using the formula for mouthwash, below.

The hospital where you work prepares a mouthwash for patients with stomatitis (mouth sores) called "magic mouthwash" that contains the following:

Hydrocortisone 100 mg/2 mL	2 mL
Nystatin suspension	30 mL
Viscous lidocaine 2%	50 mL
Diphenhydramine elixir 12.5 mg/5 mL	q.s a.d 240 mL

4. The pharmacist asks you to make 180 mL instead of 240 mL. By what factor will you reduce each ingredient to make the desired 180 mL?

5. How much diphenhydramine elixir is necessary for the original formula?

6. How much of each ingredient will be used to make 180 mL of "magic mouthwash"?

7. The children's hospital where you work dilutes heparin flush 100 units/mL in normal saline for injection to make a special low-dose heparin flush syringe for newborns. The low-dose solution contains 1 unit heparin/mL and each syringe contains 0.5 mL. Your boss asks you to make 50 of these syringes.
   a. How much heparin is contained in 50 of the low-dose heparin flush syringes?
   b. How much of the heparin 100 units/mL will you use to make the dilute flush solution?
   c. How much normal saline for injection will you add to the heparin in Part b to make the dilute heparin flush solution?

8. You need to measure 125 mg magnesium sulfate for a product you are compounding. The sensitivity rating of the balance is 10 mg and there is an acceptable error rate of 4%.
   a. What is the minimum weighable quantity for the magnesium sulfate?
   b. You are to dilute the magnesium sulfate with equal parts lactose powder. The pharmacist-in-charge tells you to make 500 mg of the mixture of magnesium sulfate and lactose. How much lactose will you need?

c. What aliquot will you measure out to contain the desired amount (125 mg) of magnesium sulfate?

9. The sensitivity rating of your balance is 6 mg and the acceptable error rate is 3.5%. What is the minimum weighable quantity?

10. Find the minimum weighable quantity for the following:
    a. Sensitivity rating = 4 mg, permissible error 4%
    b. Sensitivity rating = 2 mg, acceptable error rate 5%

11. In the pediatrics unit of your hospital, a physician orders morphine for a patient who has undergone surgery and is in pain. The morphine is to be drawn up into a 10-mL syringe and administered via a pump that can deliver as little as 0.5 mL/hr. The orders are for morphine 0.25 mg per hour with instruction for the nurse to increase the dose as needed to a maximum of 0.75 mg per hour. The pharmacist tells you to use 10 mg/mL morphine diluted with normal saline to make 10 mL of morphine 0.5 mg/mL.
    a. How much morphine is contained in 10 mL of morphine 0.5 mg/mL?
    b. How much of the morphine 10 mg/mL is needed to make the dilute solution?
    c. How much normal saline will be used to make the dilute solution?
    d. What volume of the dilute solution contains 0.25 mg of morphine?

12. A veterinarian orders a solution that contains 10 mg of an antibiotic in 20 mL of solution. The balance in the pharmacy has a sensitivity rating of 5 mg and the allowable error is 4%.
    a. What is the minimum weighable quantity?
    b. What total volume of solution will be needed to make the necessary final concentration?

13. An antacid product contains 650 mg calcium carbonate and 500 mg sorbitol in each tablet. Each bottle contains 120 tablets. How much of each ingredient is needed to make 1000 bottles?

14. The density of a correctly compounded IV solution is 1.01 g/mL at room temperature. You will dispense 1 liter of the solution in an IV bag that, when empty, has a mass of 121 g.
    a. What is the mass of 1 liter of the solution?
    b. What will the bag and the solution weigh together?

15. The density of mineral oil at 15°C is 0.76 g/mL and the density of water at the same temperature is 0.99 g/mL. What is the specific gravity of mineral oil?

16. The volume of drug A is 15 mL and the weight is 16 grams. What is the density of drug A?

17. You measure out 32 grams of anhydrous ferrous sulfate, which has a density of 2.8 g/cm³. What volume will this amount of ferrous sulfate fill?

18. In the pharmacy technology laboratory, Mary weighs out 260 mg of acetylsalicylic acid powder. Her lab partner Diane reweighs the powder on the more accurate electronic balance and finds the weight of the powder to be 264 mg. What is the percent error of the less accurate balance?

19. Jocelyn uses a graduated cylinder to measure 45 mL of an oral solution. The pharmacist tells her to draw the solution up in a 60-mL syringe instead, because it will be more accurate. When she draws the solution up into the syringe, she sees that the volume is 42 mL.

    a. What could account for the shortage?
    b. Assuming that all the solution made it into the syringe, what is the percent error of the graduated cylinder Jocelyn originally used?

20. A solution weighs 84 g and fills a 100-mL vial. What is its density?

21. At room temperature, 99% ethanol has a density of 0.83 g/mL. You have an 8 fluid ounce and a pint bottle. Which bottle will you choose to hold 265 g of ethanol?

22. You are asked to make Dakin's ½ strength solution for a patient with a wound. The formula calls for 952 mL sterile water for irrigation and 48 mL sodium hypochlorite 5.25% solution (bleach) and you need 250 mL for the day.

    a. How much Dakin's ½ strength does the formula make?
    b. How much of each ingredient do you need to make 250 mL of the solution?

23. The dermatologist orders the following ointment frequently for her patients with seborrheic dermatitis:

Precipitated sulfur	10 g
salicylic acid	2.5 g
water soluble ointment base	qs to 100 g

    a. How much of each ingredient is needed to make 1 kg of ointment?
    b. How much of each ingredient is necessary to make 454 grams?

24. Al Aiken brings in a prescription for 6 oz of the wintergreen sports rub shown in Figure 12-1.

    a. By what factor will the weight of each ingredient be multiplied to make 6 oz of the sports rub?
    b. How much of each ingredient is needed to make 6 oz?

25. The density of corn oil at room temperature is 0.92 g/mL. Of a quart, pint, and half-gallon capacity bottle, which would best contain the volume of 1 kg of corn oil?

CHAPTER 13

IV Infusions and Injectable Drugs

LEARNING OBJECTIVES

1. Determine the amount of a drug in a vial or bottle, the volume the dry powder displaces, and the concentration of the drug when incorrectly reconstituted.

2. Define *milliequivalent* (mEq), and convert a measurement from milliequivalents to milligrams.

3. Define *millimole (mM)* and convert a measurement from millimole to mg.

4. Given an infusion rate, calculate the delivery time for a specified volume of fluid.

UNIT 4

Introduction

One of the most crucial aspects of the pharmacy technician's work in a hospital setting is centered on sterile compounding. This work is crucial because the compounded products are delivered directly into the patient's blood stream and cannot be removed once administered. If an error in calculations is made, the product is contaminated, or the wrong drug is selected, the patient, family, and pharmacy staff must deal with the results of the error. The rule of thumb in pharmacy compounding, especially sterile compounding, is that if a technician suspects that contamination occurred or an error was made while compounding, throw out the product and start over.

> ### TECH NOTE!
>
> *In the pharmacy, "when in doubt, throw it out" means never dispense a product to a patient if you suspect an error was made in compounding.*

Products for injection are typically more expensive than products for oral use, because they are manufactured in more controlled settings to assure sterility. Although it is far better to waste an incorrectly made sterile product than administer it to the patient, the meticulous technician will avoid costly errors by checking and double-checking calculations before beginning. In this chapter you will learn about the calculations and units frequently used when preparing sterile compounds and other preparations.

Reconstituting Medications

Whether in retail or institutional pharmacy workplaces, pharmacy technicians reconstitute medications. When a medication is **reconstituted**, it is brought to a liquid state by the addition of water or another diluent, such as normal saline. Drugs that require reconstitution generally have a short shelf-life as liquid preparations,

Reconstitute—To bring a medication to the liquid state by the addition of water or another diluent.

so to avoid unnecessary waste, they are usually reconstituted immediately prior to use. Examples include both oral and injectable antibiotic preparations, chemotherapeutic agents, and some injectable hormone preparations.

Usually reconstitution is a straightforward process. The label or package insert contains the information necessary to successfully reconstitute any dry preparation. It is possible to make mistakes when reconstituting a medication, however. If the product involved costs just a few dollars, most pharmacists would instruct the technician to waste the incorrectly prepared product and start again. Unfortunately, there are many preparations that cost hundreds or even thousands of dollars. When an expensive product can be salvaged through knowledge of the mathematics involved, sharp technicians may be saving their jobs as well!

There is no way to undo mixing a medication with an incompatible solution, so be extra careful to select the correct diluent before mixing. When an incorrect volume of the right diluent is used for reconstitution, the error does not necessarily render the product unusable. Obviously, if too little diluent is used, the difference can be added to correct the problem. If too much diluent is added, it clearly cannot be removed. For some uses, such as subcutaneous or intramuscular injection where the maximum volume that can be injected is limited, this will likely result in wasting the product. However, for oral or intravenous use, if the new concentration can be calculated, the diluted product might still be fit for use. The question is, how do you determine the new concentration? Remember, concentration of a reconstituted liquid is written as units of mass/units of volume. If you know the amount of the drug in the vial and the volume it occupies, and the volume of the added diluent is known, it is possible to determine the new concentration of the product. Study the examples below to learn this process.

EXAMPLE

After reconstitution with 117 mL water, a bottle of amoxicillin 250 mg/5 mL contains 150 mL suspension for oral administration. What volume does the dry powder displace before reconstitution?

SOLUTION

Since the volume of the fluid after reconstitution is known and the volume of added diluent is known, you can determine the volume the dry powder displaces by subtraction.

150 mL final volume − 117 mL water added = 33 mL powder displacement volume

EXAMPLE

Clarithromycin for oral suspension is supplied as a powder that when reconstituted contains clarithromycin 125 mg/5 mL. How much clarithromycin (in mg) is in a 50-mL bottle?

SOLUTION

You can use dimensional analysis to answer this question.

125 mg/5 mL × 50 mL/bottle = 1250 mg/bottle

EXAMPLE

Patsy, the P.T. at St. Madeleine's Hospital, was reconstituting a multidose vial of Fortaz® injection to make IV piggyback bags. The label directed Patsy to add 26 mL to the Fortaz® vial to make 30 mL of ceftazidime 1 gram/5 mL. She realized, too late, that she added 36 mL water instead. The pharmacist said that a multidose vial of Fortaz® is expensive, and asked Patsy to figure out the new concentration rather than waste the vial.

SOLUTION ···

First, Patsy calculated the amount of ceftazidime in the vial. She knew that the correctly reconstituted solution contains 30 mL of ceftazidime 1 g/5 mL. She did not remove any drug from the container, so the amount (in g) of drug when correctly reconstituted was the same amount as in the incorrectly reconstituted product.

$$1 \text{ g/5 mL} \times 30 \text{ mL} = 6 \text{ g of ceftazidime}$$

Next, Patsy calculated the volume the powder in the container displaces.

30 mL (correct final volume) – 26 mL (added water) = 4 mL dry powder volume

Patsy calculated the final volume of the incorrectly reconstituted medication by adding the volume of the dry powder to the volume of water she used.

4 mL (dry powder) + 36 mL (added water) = 40 mL final volume

Finally, Patsy calculated the concentration of the incorrectly reconstituted medication.

6 g ceftazidime/40 mL = 0.15 g/ mL

In order to make 1 g ceftazidime IV piggybacks, what volume of this solution is needed? Patsy used a ratio and proportion equation to calculate the new volume.

$$\frac{0.15 \text{ g}}{1 \text{ mL}} = \frac{1 \text{ g}}{x}$$

$$1 \text{ g} (1 \text{ mL}) = 0.15 \text{ g} (x)$$

$$x = \frac{1 \text{ mL}}{0.15} = 6.7 \text{ mL contains 1 g}$$

Milliequivalents and Millimoles

So far, you have learned about a number of different ways of measuring substances. Pharmacy technicians also need to know about a couple of other units of measurement that always come up in discussions about sterile compounding. If you have taken a general chemistry course, these units may already be familiar.

Electrolytes are minerals that, when dissolved in liquid, carry an electrical charge. The charged particles are called ions. Electrolytes are essential to normal physiologic function in the body, where their movement in and out of cells allows

Electrolytes—A chemical compound that can conduct electrical current.

muscles to contract and nerves to carry impulses, among other actions. Some of the electrolytes most important to these physiologic actions include sodium, potassium, calcium, phosphate, and magnesium. People normally take electrolytes in through their diet. However, if a person is taking medications or has a condition that causes depletion of electrolytes, or is unable to take food and beverages by mouth, these electrolytes must be replaced in order to maintain or restore normal balances.

Electrolyte concentrations are typically expressed in units of milliequivalents or millimoles. A mole is a unit of measurement used in chemistry. The mass (commonly referred to as weight) of one mole of an element, expressed in grams, is equal to that substance's atomic weight as listed on the periodic table of the elements. Table 13-1 shows atomic weights of some commonly used electrolytes. When the atomic weight is expressed as milligrams, it equals one one thousandth of a mole, or a **millimole**.

Millimole—One thousandth of a mole.

Table 13-1. Molecular Formulas and mEq Weights for Commonly Used Electrolytes

Molecular Formula	Atomic Weight of Components	Molecular Weight	Valence	1 mEq Weight
$NaCl$	Sodium 23, Chloride 35.5	58.5	1	58.5 mg
KCl	Potassium 39, Chloride 35.5	74.5	1	74.5 mg
$NaC_2H_3O_2$	Sodium 23, Acetate 59	84	1	84 mg
$MgSO_4$	Magnesium 24, Sulphate 96, $(H_2O)_7$	246	2	123 mg
$CaCl_2$	Calcium 40, Chloride 71, $(H_2O)_2$	147	2	73.5 mg
$NaHCO_3$	Sodium 23, Bicarbonate 61	84	1	84 mg

EXAMPLE

How much does one mole (M) of sodium weigh?

SOLUTION ···

The atomic weight of sodium is 22.9898. In a typical pharmacy-related problem this weight would be rounded; so one mole of sodium weighs 23 g.

EXAMPLE

How much would one millimole (mM) of sodium chloride weigh?

SOLUTION ···

The weight of one mole or millimole of a molecule would be calculated in the same way that a mole or millimole of an atom is determined. We know that a millimole of sodium would weigh 23 mg. The atomic weight of chloride is 35.5. To determine the weight of the molecule NaCl, the weight of each component is added together.

23 mg (one mM Na) + 35.5 mg (one mM Cl) = 58.5 milligrams (one mM NaCl)

When sodium chloride is dissolved in a liquid, the sodium and chloride atoms separate into positively charged (sodium) and negatively charged (chloride) ions. Notice that in the equation above, one millimole of the molecule sodium chloride yields one millimole of each electrolyte when dissolved. In a stable molecule, the positive and negative charges will always add up to zero. That means that an ion that carries two positive charges will combine with a particle or particles that carry two negative charges so that the total charge is zero.

Valence and equivalent weights

The **valence** of an element represents its capacity to combine with other elements to form stable molecules. An element can have different valence numbers, because it can exist in different forms. Valence is important because equivalent weights are based on valence. One milliequivalent of a molecule is equal to its molecular weight expressed as milligrams (or one mM) divided by its valence.

$$1 \text{ mEq} = \frac{\text{molecular weight in mg (1 mM)}}{\text{valence}}$$

This is not as straightforward as it looks, because molecules often occur in different forms, so using valence to arrive at the milliequivalent weight of a molecule can be confusing. To simplify, just use Table 13-1 (or other reference tables) to find milliequivalent weights for commonly used electrolyte solutions. In addition, this information is available on the labels of electrolyte vials, as seen in Figure 13-1. Sometimes you will need to convert between milliequivalents and milligrams. If you divide a given weight of a substance by its milliequivalent weight, the result is the number of milliequivalents. Try working the following problems without looking at the answers to test your understanding of these concepts.

Valence—The capacity of an element to combine with other elements, compared with that of one hydrogen atom.

UNIT **4**

Figure 13-1. Labels on electrolyte vials contain concentrations in milliequivalents and weight.

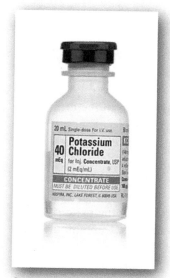

Source: Reprinted with permission of Hospira, Inc.

EXAMPLE

After the lab results show that Sally Eine's sodium levels are low, the physician asks that an additional 40 mEq of sodium chloride be added to her TPN. You have 23.4% sodium chloride concentrate available. How much of this concentrated solution contains 40 mEq?

SOLUTION ···

From the table you can see that 1 mEq of NaCl weighs 58.5 mg, so

$$\frac{58.5 \text{ mg}}{1 \text{ mEq}} \times 40 \text{ mEq} = 2340 \text{ mg} = 2.34 \text{ g}$$

A 23.4% solution contains 23.4 g/100 mL. If 23.4 g is contained in 100 mL, then 2.34 g (one tenth) will be contained in 10 mL. So, 10 mL NaCl concentrate will contain the ordered 40 mEq NaCl.

EXAMPLE

Cal Imiya brings in prescriptions for hydrochlorothiazide 25 mg tablets and KCl 20% elixir. The physician has ordered 20 mEq of KCl to be given twice daily. Calculate the volume that will contain 20 mEq of KCl.

SOLUTION ···

By definition, a 20% KCl elixir contains 20g KCl/100 mL. Table 13-1 indicates that the molecular weight of KCl is 74.5 and the valence is one, so 1 milliequivalent = 74.5 mg, and 20 mEq = 1490 mg or 1.49 g. Now use a ratio and proportion equation to determine the volume needed to deliver 1.49 g.

$$20 \text{ g}/100 \text{ mL} = 1.49 \text{ g}/x$$

$$x = \frac{149 \text{ g (mL)}}{20 \text{ g}} = 7.45 \text{ mL, rounded to 7.5 mL}$$

Intravenous Infusion Flow Rates

All products sent to patient care areas for intravenous infusion are labeled with the contents of the container and directions regarding the rate of infusion or the "flow rate." This infusion rate is comparable to the signa on a prescription for oral use, and directs the person giving the medication on how to set up the infusion.

For large volume parenteral medications, such as fluid and electrolyte replacement products, the physician will include the desired flow rate in the drug order. The flow rate of total parenteral nutrition is determined by the physician, in consultation with the pharmacist or dietitian, or with the use of protocols or guidelines.

When the infusion rate and volume of an ordered product is known, the pharmacy technician can easily calculate the length of time it will take for the product to be infused. This has a bearing on how many IV bags are made for any specified period of time or how frequently medications are resupplied to the patient, which is important information for the technician working in the IV compounding area.

Infusion rates are usually expressed as mL/hour. However, sometimes IV drips are ordered based on the medication dissolved in the solution. For example, a morphine drip would be ordered as milligrams of morphine infused per hour. Either way, the volume infused each hour can be calculated. Then, because the total volume of the IV bag is known, the period of time over which the bag will infuse can be calculated.

EXAMPLE

Dr. Annie Watters ordered an IV for Les Dryer. She wants the IV to run at 150 mL/hr × 4 hours, and then the rate is to be reduced to 100 mL/hr. The ordered IV solution is available in 1000-mL bags. How many will you send to meet Mr. Dryer's needs for 24 hours?

SOLUTION

First, calculate the volume of fluid infused in the initial 4 hours.

$$\frac{150 \text{ mL}}{\text{hr}} \times 4 \text{ hr} = 600 \text{ mL}$$

Next, calculate the amount of fluid required for the next 20 hours.

$$\frac{100 \text{ mL}}{\text{hr}} \times 20 \text{ hr} = 2000 \text{ mL}$$

Now, the volumes are totaled and divided by the volume in one bag to determine the number of IV bags to deliver to the patient care area.

$$200 \text{ mL} + 600 \text{ mL} = 2600 \text{ mL}$$

$$\frac{2600 \text{ mL}}{1000 \text{ mL}} = 2.6 \text{ bags}$$

Clearly, there is no way to send 0.6 bags, so the only option is to send 3 bags of the ordered IV fluid.

EXAMPLE

If the first IV bag for Les Dryer is hung at 1500 hours, what time will the next IV bag be due?

SOLUTION

Mr. Dryer's IV bags contain 1000 mL each. As previously calculated, 600 mL of the bag will infuse in 4 hours. The 400 mL remaining infuse at a rate of 100 mL/hr, so they will run in over another 4 hours, for a total of 8 hours for the first bag.

Therefore, the next bag is due at 1500 hours + 8 hours = 2300 hours, or 11:00 PM

EXAMPLE

It is change of shift at Mercy Hospital. You receive a telephone call from Watson Watts, R.N. for a refill on a 1mg/ mL morphine drip for a patient. "You need this already? I just sent a bag a few hours ago," you say. He replies that the new bag was hung 3 hours ago, but the patient receives 5 mg/hr and he wants to make certain the replacement is available when needed. If the morphine drip provided contained 100 mL, how much is left in the bag, and how long will it last?

SOLUTION ··

The bag is infusing at a rate of 5 mg/hr and every mL contains 1 mg of morphine. Calculate the infusion rate using dimensional analysis.

$$\frac{1 \text{ mL}}{\text{mg}} \times \frac{5 \text{ mg}}{\text{hr}} = 5 \text{ mL}\bigg/\text{hr}$$

You know that when full, the bag contains 100 mL. How long would a full IV bag last?

$$100 \text{ mL} \times 1 \text{ hr}/5 \text{ mL} = 20 \text{ hours}$$

At this rate, a full bag will run for 20 hours. The bag has already been infusing for 3 hours so there are 17 hours worth of medication left in the IV bag. It would be appropriate to call Watson back and let him know that the IV should last through the entire shift.

EXAMPLE

Nurse Barbie Kuan is hungry and has to hang an IV piggy back before she heads across the street to the park for the hospital picnic. The bag she is to hang contains 250 mL of fluid plus a small volume of medication. She's hoping to start the infusion, go eat, and make it back before the bag is empty. The label says to infuse at a rate of 170 mL/hr. Approximately how long will it take to infuse the solution?

SOLUTION ··

Use ratio and proportion or dimensional analysis to solve this problem.

$$\frac{170 \text{ mL}}{1 \text{ hr}} = \frac{250 \text{ mL}}{x}$$

$$\frac{250 \text{ mL (hr)}}{170 \text{ mL}} \approx 1.5 \text{ hr}$$

or

$$250 \text{ mL} \times \frac{1 \text{ hr}}{170 \text{ mL}} \approx 1.5 \text{ hr for the bag to run in}$$

Sometimes infusion rates might be expressed as an amount of medication per minute, instead of per hour. Whether expressed as milligrams or micrograms or milliliters per minute, multiplying by a factor of 60 min/hr allows for conversion to an hourly rate.

EXAMPLE

Dr. Harte orders a dopamine drip to run at 60 mcg/min for a baby in the pediatric ICU. The pharmacist asks you to make up a 25-mL dopamine syringe with a concentration of 1600 mcg/ mL. How long will the syringe last?

SOLUTION ··

To convert the rate from mcg/min to mcg/hr, multiply by 60 min/hr.

$$\frac{60 \text{ mcg}}{\text{min}} \times \frac{60 \text{ min}}{\text{hr}} = 3600 \text{ mcg/hr}$$

The solution contains 1600 mcg/mL. To determine the number of mL that will infuse over 1 hour, first use a ratio and proportion equation to find out how many mL contain 3600 mcg.

$$\frac{1600 \text{ mcg}}{1 \text{ mL}} = \frac{3600 \text{ mcg}}{x}$$

x = 3600 mcg (1 mL)/1600 mcg = 2.25 mL, which contains 3600 mcg

Therefore, the syringe will run in at a rate of 2.25 mL/hr. The volume of the syringe is 25 mL. Using dimensional analysis we see that:

$$25 \text{ mL} \times 1 \text{ hr}/2.25 \text{ mL} = \text{about 11 hours}$$

Infusion pumps

Before the advent of automated pumps that control rates of infusions, different caliber infusion sets were used to manage infusion rates. If a nurse used an IV set that delivered 60 drops for every mL of fluid, he or she could make finer adjustments to the infusion rate than an infusion set that delivered only 20 drops for every mL of fluid. If the rate, in drops per minute, and the number of drops per mL delivered was known, then the flow rate could be calculated.

EXAMPLE

Nurse Betty hung an IV using an infusion set that delivered 60 drops for every mL of fluid infused. The drip rate was 30 gtts/min. What was the infusion rate in mL/hr?

SOLUTION

You can use dimensional analysis to convert drops per minute to mL/minute and then to mL/hr as follows:

$$\frac{30 \text{ gtts}}{\text{min}} \times \frac{1 \text{ mL}}{60 \text{ gtts}} \times \frac{60 \text{ min}}{\text{hr}} = 30 \text{ mL/hr}$$

No matter what the size of the IV set, this same problem-solving approach could be used to convert drip rates to mL/hr.

Fortunately, nearly every hospital now uses automated infusion pumps. For this kind of equipment, the nurse programs the flow rate into the pump. Only one type of tubing is necessary, and depending on the pump, a wide range of infusion rates is possible. Some "smart" IV pumps even warn the nurse about dangerous drug doses or infusion rates (see Figure 13-2).

Figure 13-2. An automated IV smart pump.

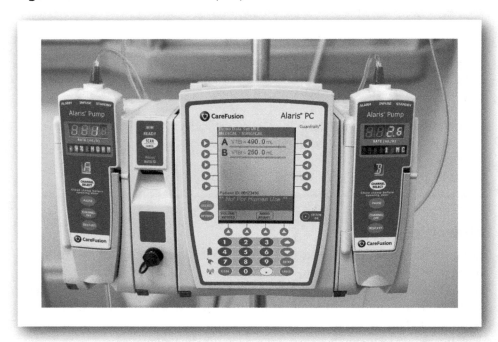

Source: Reprinted with permission of CareFusion.

Practice Problems

1. A vial of cefazolin for IV use is reconstituted with 45 mL of fluid and contains 50 mL of cefazolin 1 g/5 mL when correctly reconstituted.
   a. What volume does the dry powder displace?
   b. How many grams of cefazolin are in the vial?
   c. To prepare a 2-g dose, what volume will be withdrawn?

2. Gwen Tuphaz, P.T., prepared the above vial using 65 mL of fluid instead of 45 mL.
   a. What is the concentration of the incorrectly prepared cefazolin?
   b. What volume contains the desired 2-g dose?

3. The pharmacist prepares amoxicillin oral suspension that contains 500 mg/5 mL when correctly reconstituted. A full bottle contains 150 mL. How much amoxicillin is in a full bottle?

4. A ceftriaxone vial directs you to add 3.6 mL of fluid to a 1-gram vial. The resulting solution contains 250 mg/mL.
   a. What is the total volume in the reconstituted vial?
   b. What volume does the dry powder displace?

5. Nurse Nancy calls you from the surgery unit to say that she mistakenly read the ceftriaxone reconstitution directions and added 5.6 mL lidocaine 1% instead of 3.6 mL. She is a new graduate and asks you what she should do. The ceftriaxone is for an IM injection in a woman who weighs 50 kg. You answer (choose the best answer):
   a. "I'm not certain. Let me look into it and call you back."
   b. "Let me get the pharmacist for you. Will you please hold?"
   c. "This medication is inexpensive, and it would be uncomfortable to inject 6 mL of fluid. I suggest you throw it away and start over."

6. The directions for reconstitution of pantoprazole 40 mg for IV use state the vial is to be reconstituted with normal saline, but you just reconstituted it with a 5% dextrose solution. Should you use it anyway? Why or why not?

7. You receive a drug order for 5% dextrose in water 1000 mL, plus 30 mEq KCl. A vial of KCl contains 2 mEq KCl/mL. What volume of KCl will you add to the 1000-mL bag?

8. While working at ABC Pediatric Pharmacy, you mistakenly reconstitute cephalexin for 100-mL oral suspension with 96 mL of water instead of 71. When correctly reconstituted, the suspension contains 250 mg/5 mL cephalexin.
   a. How much cephalexin does the bottle contain?
   b. How much volume does the powder displace?
   c. What is the concentration of the incorrectly reconstituted suspension?
   d. What volume of the incorrectly mixed product contains 250 mg?

9. Normal saline contains 0.9% NaCl. How many mEq of sodium are there in a 100-mL bag of normal saline? Refer to Table 13-1 for equivalent weight of sodium chloride.

10. Sodium chloride is available in 1-g tablets. How many milliequivalents of sodium are in 1 tablet?

11. A patient receives one 50-mEq prefilled syringe of sodium bicarbonate IV during a code blue. One mEq of sodium bicarbonate weighs 84 mg. How many grams of sodium bicarbonate did the patient receive?

12. A physician prescribes KCl 8-mEq tablets to be given three times a day. Unfortunately, only 10% KCl liquid is covered by the patient's insurance. The pharmacist gets the okay for a switch to liquid, but wants you to calculate the dose for her to check. See Table 13-1.
    a. How many mL of 10% KCl contain 8 mEq?
    b. The patient must dilute KCl before drinking it. Usually, 20 mEq is mixed in 4 ounces of juice or water. To mix 8 mEq in the same concentration, with what volume of juice or water will it be mixed?

13. Prefilled sodium bicarbonate syringes, made especially to use in cardiac and respiratory emergencies for infants and young children, contain 10 mL of 4.2% sodium bicarbonate.
    a. How many mEq of sodium bicarbonate are in a syringe?
    b. How many mEq of sodium bicarbonate are in 1 mL of the solution?

14. The directions on all of the following IVPB bags indicate they should run in at a rate of 200 mL/hr. How long will each bag last?
    a. 50 mL IVPB
    b. 100 mL IVPB
    c. 150 mL IVPB
    d. 200 mL IVPB

15. A physician orders that a patient receive 3000 mL of TPN fluids in a day.
    a. How many mL/hr will the patient receive?
    b. The orders for the TPN are received and processed at 1700 hours. The next batch of IV solutions will be made in the morning and delivered at 0900 hours. How many bags will the technician need to make to last until morning?

16. At Little Hospital, near Tiny Town, Texas, the 40-bed hospital owns 6 IV pumps. If a seventh patient needs an IV, the nurses use drip rates to set the infusion rate. The IV set delivers 20 gtts/mL, and the IV needs to run at 60 mL/hr.
    a. How many drops per hour will the patient receive?
    b. How many drops per minute will provide 60 mL/hr?

17. The physician orders a 500-mL bag of fluid to run in over 4 hours. How many mL/minute will the patient receive?

18. The standard magnesium sulfate bags for obstetrics contain 20 g $MgSO_4$/500 mL of fluid. The order you receive for Mrs. Bertha Cummins for her pre-term labor are as follows:

    Initiate treatment with 4 g $MgSO_4$ to run in over 30 minutes. Follow with magnesium sulfate 2 g per hour.
    a. How many mL will contain the initial dose of 4 g?
    b. How long will the first 500-mL bag last?
    c. How long will subsequent 500-mL bags last?

19. The ICU pharmacist calls the central pharmacy to get a dopamine drip made for a patient. The standard concentration for dopamine drips in your hospital is 1600 mcg/mL. Dopamine is available as 40 mg/mL in a 5-mL vial. How much dopamine will you add to a 250-mL bag to achieve the standard concentration?

20. A few hours after you made the dopamine bag in Problem 19, the ICU pharmacist calls down to say the patient is getting worse. The pharmacist asks for a double concentration of the dopamine in a 100-mL bag. He asks you to bring the mixed bag, with your calculations, right away because the patient is critically ill.

    a. How much dopamine will you add to 100 mL normal saline to make twice the concentration in Problem 19?

    b. If the double concentration bag is set to run at 400 mcg/min, how long will a 100-mL bag last?

21. A stat IV order is written for a dehydrated patient. The order reads "1000 mL NS + 20 KCl, run in over 4 hours, then 150 mL/hr for 6 hours, then 125 mL/hr." After 6 hours the above orders are discontinued. How much normal saline has the patient received after 6 hours?

22. The new orders for the patient in Problem 21 call for KCl 60 mEq/1000 mL NS. A vial of KCl contains 2 mEq/mL. How many mL of KCl will be added to the new bag?

23. The home health pharmacy prepares peripheral nutrition bags for 83-year-old Leanne Abed, who is recovering from burns she sustained when her kitchen caught fire. The IV infuses at a rate of 100 mL/hr. Mrs. Abed also receives antibiotics at midnight, 0600, 1200, and 1800. The TPN is turned off for 30 minutes every 6 hours while the antibiotics infuse. How much TPN does Mrs. Abed receive in 1 day?

24. The pharmacy usually delivers Mrs. Abed's IV bags at noon, but today the delivery truck broke down. Her last bag was hung at 0700, and delivery is anticipated at 1800. Will she have enough fluid in the bag to keep it running until 1800?

25. Insulin drips are used to treat a serious condition in patients with poorly controlled diabetes, called diabetic ketoacidosis. In your hospital, the standard concentration of an insulin drip is 1 unit/mL in 100-mL bags. Patient Annie Sweet is in the ICU and an insulin drip is ordered. Annie receives 8 units/hr for 4 hours, then 6 units/hr for 3 hours, and for the last 7 hours has received 5 units/hour. How much fluid is left in Annie's IV bag?

CHAPTER 14

Business Math

LEARNING OBJECTIVES

1. Calculate markup, gross profit, net profit, and discount.
2. Explain the concepts of average wholesale price and insurance reimbursement.
3. Calculate inventory turnover.
4. Find the annual depreciation of a long-term asset given the initial value, the disposal value, and the estimated life of the asset.

Introduction

A pharmacy is like any other business; it must take in more money than it pays out in order to stay in business. Money paid out is the expense of running the business and can include overhead (rent, utilities), salaries, and cost to purchase and package drugs. Money taken in is known as **receipts**, or **revenue**. In hospitals or other institutional pharmacy settings, this comes from the selling price for filled drug orders, most often in the form of reimbursements from insurance companies. In retail pharmacies, prescription sales, and the merchandise from the front of the store, including over-the-counter medications and health and beauty products, are the sources of revenue. The difference between receipts and expenses is called profit. Receipts must be greater than expenses for the pharmacy to make a profit. Often times the difference between a successful business and one that fails is a matter of keeping costs down by avoiding waste and making cost-effective purchasing decisions.

Receipts—The amount of money received.

Revenue—The total of all money received from the sale of a firm's product or service during a given period.

> ▶ **TECH NOTE!**
>
> *Profit is dependent upon keeping costs lower than revenue.*

Markup, Gross Profit, and Net Profit

In order to maintain a profit, pharmacies buy products at one price and sell them at a higher price. The mark-up or **gross profit** is the difference between the selling price and the purchase price. Markup rate is the ratio of markup to purchase price expressed as a percent.

Gross Profit—A business' revenue minus its cost of goods sold.

> **EXAMPLE**
>
> Joe's Pharmacy buys 20-mg Ritalin® tablets for $64.00 for a bottle of 30 tablets. Joe fills a prescription for Miss Anita Focus for 30 tablets and charges her $75.00. What is the markup on this prescription?

SOLUTION ···

Purchase price = $64.00
Selling price = $75.00
Markup = purchase price – selling price
Markup = $75.00 – $64.00 = $11.00

EXAMPLE

Joe's Pharmacy buys a 6-ounce bottle of Caladryl® Lotion for $3.50. Joe sells the bottle to Boyd Seechan for $7.00. What is the markup rate on the Caladryl®?

SOLUTION ···

Purchase price = $3.50
Selling price = $7.00
Markup = selling price – purchase price
Markup = $7.00 – $3.50 = $3.50
Markup rate = (markup/purchase price) × 100%

Markup rate = $\dfrac{3.50}{3.50}$ × 100% = 100%

EXAMPLE

Joe's Pharmacy buys a bottle of 30 Ambien® CR 12.5-mg tablets for $190.00.

Ms. Ivana Dozoff has a prescription for 30 Ambien® CR tablets. Joe's markup rate on this drug is 45%. Find the markup. Find the price Ms. Dozoff is charged.

SOLUTION ···

Markup = markup rate × purchase price
Markup = 0.45 × 190.00
Markup = $85.50
Selling price = purchase price + markup
Selling price = $190.00 + $85.50 = $275.50

Discount

Pharmacies and suppliers may offer a product at a price lower than the regular price. The difference between the regular price and the lower price is called the **discount**.

Discount— A reduction from the full or standard amount of a price.

EXAMPLE

The regular price of amoxapine 50 mg is $63.00 for 90 tablets. One supplier sells them at a discounted price of $50.00 for 90 tablets. What is the amount of the discount?

SOLUTION ·····································

Discount = regular price – selling price

Discount = $63.00 – $50.00 = $13.00

When the discount is given as a percent of the regular price, this is called the **discount rate**.

UNIT 4

EXAMPLE

Geodon® 40 mg tablets regularly sell for $180.00 for 60 tablets. A supplier is offering a one-time 14% discount on Geodon® 40-mg tablets. What is the discount and the selling price for 60 Geodon® 40-mg tablets?

SOLUTION ···

Discount = discount rate × regular price

Discount = 0.14 × $180.00 = $25.20

Selling price = regular price – discount

Selling price = $180.00 – $25.20 = $154.80

EXAMPLE

The regular price for 36 Sinutab® sinus and allergy tablets is $9.15. Joe's Pharmacy is selling these at a 15% discount. What is the discounted selling price?

SOLUTION ···

Discount = discount rate × regular price

Discount = 0.15 × $9.15 = $1.37

Selling price = regular price – discount

Selling price = $9.15 – $1.37 = $7.78

Average Wholesale Price

Pharmacies are seldom paid directly by the patient for the entire cost of a prescription medication. Most of the time, the patient's insurance company reimburses the pharmacy. The amount that an insurance company will reimburse for a given drug is based on the **average wholesale price (AWP)** of that drug. The average wholesale price for any drug is the average price that wholesalers charge pharmacies for the drug. Generally the insurance company will reimburse the pharmacy at a set percentage of AWP plus a set dispensing fee. Some insurers will pay based on acquisition cost plus a dispensing fee. The farther below AWP the pharmacy can purchase drugs, the greater the profit will be.

EXAMPLE

The AWP for 88 mcg levothyroxine is $33.00 for 90 tablets. Joe's pharmacy purchases 90 tablets for $30.00. Mattie Bolich fills her prescription for 90 tablets at Joe's. Her insurance company reimburses the pharmacy at AWP plus 5% plus a $4.00 dispensing fee. How much profit does Joe's make in filling this prescription?

SOLUTION ···

First calculate the amount of the reimbursement.

0.05($33.00) = $1.65

Reimbursement = $33.00 + $1.65 + $4.00 = $38.65

Gross profit = $38.65 − $30.00 = $8.65

Inventory

Inventory Value—The value of goods held.

Pharmacies need to maintain an accurate inventory, which is a list of items in the pharmacy available to sell. **Inventory value** is the worth of all those items on a given day. Keeping medication on the shelf for long periods means that money that could otherwise earn interest is tied up in inventory costs. On the other hand, the pharmacy must be prepared to fill prescriptions for medication that may be slow moving. An accurate inventory provides information that enables staff to make informed decision on reordering drugs and keeping appropriate quantities on hand.

Some pharmacies utilize automated ordering systems that provide accurate inventory information at any time. Others may perform a physical inventory count once to several times per year. When knowledge of inventory value at multiple points in the year is available, an average inventory value can then be calculated. **Average inventory value** is calculated like any other average. The equation below shows the calculation using two values. The number in the denominator reflects the number of inventory values available:

Average Inventory Value— Sum of inventory values divided by number of inventories.

Average inventory value = (initial inventory value + current inventory value)/2

Turnover Rate—Measures the number of times a company sells its inventory during the year.

This average inventory value can then be used to determine the **turnover rate**, the number of times per year that the value of the inventory was sold.

Turnover rate = amount paid for inventory in 1 year/average inventory value

---
EXAMPLE

In January, the staff at Joe's Pharmacy performs an inventory and discovers that the value of the inventory is $65,000.00. Six months later another inventory is performed and the value is $90,000.00. Over the course of a year, Joe spends $232,500.00 purchasing items to sell at the pharmacy. Find the average inventory value and the turnover rate. How long does it take to "turn over" the inventory?

SOLUTION ···

Average inventory value = (initial inventory value + current inventory value)/2

Average inventory value = ($65,000.00 + $90,000.00)/2 = $77,500.00

Turnover rate = amount paid for inventory in 1 year/average inventory value

Turnover rate = $232,500.00/$77,500.00 = 3

The inventory turnover rate is three times per year, so it takes 4 months for the inventory to completely turn over.

Depreciation

A pharmacy holds both long-term and short-term assets. **Long-term assets** include buildings and equipment. Short-term assets are those that can be consumed or converted to cash within a year. **Short-term assets** include medication and other products. Long-term assets, such as a building or expensive equipment can lose value over time (see Figure 14-1). Annual **depreciation** is the loss in value divided by the estimated life of the equipment.

Annual depreciation = (total cost – disposal value)/estimated life

EXAMPLE

Neighborhood Pharmacy purchased a compact medical refrigerator for $978.00. The estimated life of the refrigerator is 5 years. After 5 years, its disposal value is $375.00. What is the annual depreciation of the refrigerator?

SOLUTION

Annual depreciation = (total cost – disposal value)/estimated life
Annual depreciation = ($978.00 – $375.00)/5 years
Annual depreciation = $120.60

A working knowledge of the business concepts presented here can add to your overall value as a pharmacy technician. Do the following practice problems to improve this set of skills so that you can become a valuable asset in your practice setting.

Figure 14-1. Long-term assets include expensive equipment such as automated dispensing cabinets.

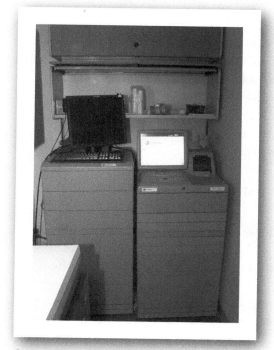

Source: Reprinted with permission of CareFusion.

Long-term Asset—Asset whose value is realized over a period of time.

Short-term Asset—Asset whose value is realized in a short period of time.

Depreciation—The loss in value divided by the estimated life of the equipment.

UNIT
4

Practice Problems

1. Joe's Pharmacy buys 30 Lipitor® 80-mg tablets for $175.00 and sells those 30 tablets for $190.00. What is Joe's gross profit on this transaction?

2. Best Pharmacy buys 4 mg Avandaryl® at $350.00 per 100 tablets. Best then sells a bottle of 60 tablets for $300.00.
   a. What does it cost Best Pharmacy to buy 60 tablets?
   b. What is Best's markup on the 60 tablets?

3. Good Neighbor Pharmacy buys 90 Naprosyn® 250-mg tablets for $16.00. Good Neighbor's markup rate on this item is 25%. What is Good Neighbor's selling price for 90 Naprosyn® 250-mg tablets?

4. Joe's Pharmacy buys fluconazole 100 mg for $350.00 for 30 tablets. It costs Joe $5.00 to dispense 30 tablets. Joe sells a bottle of 30 tablets for $435.00. What is Joe's net profit on this transaction?

5. Wholesale Rx Inc. offers Best Pharmacy a 26% discount on Effexor® 25-mg tablets. The regular wholesale price for 120 Effexor® 25-mg tablets is $270.00. What price does Best Pharmacy pay for 120 Effexor® 25-mg tablets?

6. The wholesaler, Meds R Us, offers Neighborhood Pharmacy 30 Nexium® 20-mg capsules for $165.00. The regular wholesale price for Nexium® 20-mg capsules is $195.00 for 30. What discount rate is Meds R Us offering?

7. The regular price of Lipitor® 40 mg is $98.50 for 60 tablets. Joe gets a 14% discount when buying from the wholesaler Meds R Us.
   a. What price does Joe pay for 60 tablets of Lipitor® 40 mg?
   b. It costs Joe $3.00 to dispense 60 tablets. Joe sells the 60 tablets for $95.48. What is Joe's net profit on this sale?

8. The Average Wholesale Price (AWP) for Drug D 60 mg is $150.00 for 30 tablets. Neighborhood Pharmacy can purchase Drug D 60 mg for $120.00 for 30 tablets. It costs the pharmacy $3.00 to dispense the tablets.
   a. How much does it cost Neighborhood Pharmacy to fill a prescription for 30 Drug D 60-mg tablets?
   b. The customer's insurance company will reimburse the pharmacy AWP + 4% + $4.00 dispensing fee. How much does the insurance company pay the pharmacy?
   c. What is Neighborhood Pharmacy's profit in this transaction?

9. The AWP for Actonel® 35 mg is $130.00 for 12 tablets. Joe's Pharmacy can purchase Actonel® 35 mg for $115.00 for 12 tablets. It costs the pharmacy $2.00 to dispense the tablets.
   a. How much does it cost Joe's Pharmacy to fill a prescription for 12 Actonel® 35-mg tablets?
   b. The customer's insurance company will reimburse the pharmacy AWP + 3% + $2.00 dispensing fee. How much does the insurance company pay the pharmacy?
   c. What is the pharmacy's profit in this transaction?

10. The AWP for Diovan® 160 mg is $105.00 for 84 tablets. Joe's Pharmacy can purchase Diovan® 160 mg for $100.00 for 84 tablets. It costs the pharmacy $2.00 to dispense the tablets.

   a. How much does it cost Joe's Pharmacy to fill a prescription for 84 Diovan® 160-mg tablets?

   b. The customer's insurance company will reimburse the pharmacy AWP + 4% + $5.00 dispensing fee. How much does the insurance company pay the pharmacy?

   c. What is the pharmacy's profit in this transaction?

11. The AWP for Levoxyl® 100 mcg is $54.00 for 100 tablets.

   a. What is the AWP per tablet?

   b. What is the AWP for 30 Levoxyl® 100-mcg tablets?

12. The AWP for Levoxyl® 100 mcg is $54.00 for 100 tablets. Joe's Pharmacy can purchase 90 tablets for $45.00. It costs Joe $2.00 to dispense a prescription for 30 tablets. The insurance company will reimburse AWP + 3% + $3.00 dispensing fee. What is Joe's profit in filling a prescription for 30 tablets of 100-mcg Levoxyl®?

13. In January, the staff at Joe's Pharmacy performs an inventory and discovers that the value of the inventory is $75,000.00. Six months later another inventory is performed and the value is $60,000.00. What is the average inventory?

14. In October, the staff at Neighborhood Pharmacy performs an inventory and discovers that the value of the inventory is $125,000.00. In April, another inventory is performed and the value is $99,000.00. What is the average inventory?

15. In January, the staff at Joe's Pharmacy performs an inventory and discovers that the value of the inventory is $80,000.00. Six months later another inventory is performed and the value is $100,000.00. Over the course of a year, Joe spends $360,000.00 purchasing items to sell at the pharmacy.

   a. Find the average inventory value and the turnover rate.

   b. How long does it take to "turn over" the inventory?

16. The average inventory at Neighborhood Pharmacy is $70,000.00. Over the course of a year, Neighborhood spends $210,000.00 purchasing items to sell at the pharmacy. Find the turnover rate for Neighborhood Pharmacy.

17. In January, the inventory value at Tom's Pharmacy is $125,000.00. Six months later the inventory value is $120,000.00. Over the course of a year, Tom spends $367,500.00 on items to sell. How long does it take to "turn over" the inventory at Tom's?

18. Joe's Pharmacy buys a new automatic counter for $5000.00. The expected lifetime of the equipment is 6 years. The disposal value of the counter is $2400.00. Find the annual depreciation of the automatic counter.

19. Neighborhood Pharmacy buys new compounding software for $350.00. The estimated lifetime of the software is 5 years. The disposal value of the software is $0. Find the annual depreciation for the software.

20. Tom's Pharmacy buys an electronic scale for $1075.00. The expected life of the scale is 10 years. The disposal value is $475.00. Find the annual depreciation for the scale.

21. Neighborhood Pharmacy invests in a new computer system at a cost of $12,000 for hardware and software. The life expectancy of their purchase is 6 years. The disposal value is estimated to be $750.00. Find the annual depreciation for their purchase.

22. Ralph's Pretty Good Pharmacy purchases Pretty Good Sinus Medicine for $4.54/60 and sells them for $6.81/60.
    a. What is Ralph's markup?
    b. What is Ralph's markup rate?

23. The regular wholesale price for Enditch Ointment is $5.25/ounce. Ralph buys Enditch Ointment from Prescriptions R Us for $4.00/ounce.
    a. What is the discount offered by Prescriptions R Us?
    b. What is the discount rate offered by Prescriptions R Us?

24. Medicaid reimburses Small's Pharmacy at 250% of the average acquisition cost of amoxicillin suspension plus a $4.35 professional fee. Small's pays $2.45 for a 100-mL bottle and the average acquisition cost is $2.75. It costs Bud Small $2.50 to fill the prescription.
    a. What are Bud's total costs?
    b. What does Medicaid pay Bud?
    c. What is Bud's net profit on the amoxicillin prescription?

25. Blue Shield reimburses Small's Pharmacy AWP plus a $7.50 professional fee for filling a generic prescription. The AWP for 100 furosemide 40-mg tablets is $17.80. Bud buys 100 furosemide tablets for $14.90, and his costs for filling the prescription is $3.25.
    a. What is Bud's profit when a patient has Blue Shield Insurance?
    b. Bud usually sells 100 furosemide tablets for $24.50. How much less is Bud's profit than in Part a?

Appendices

Appendix A—Parts of a Prescription

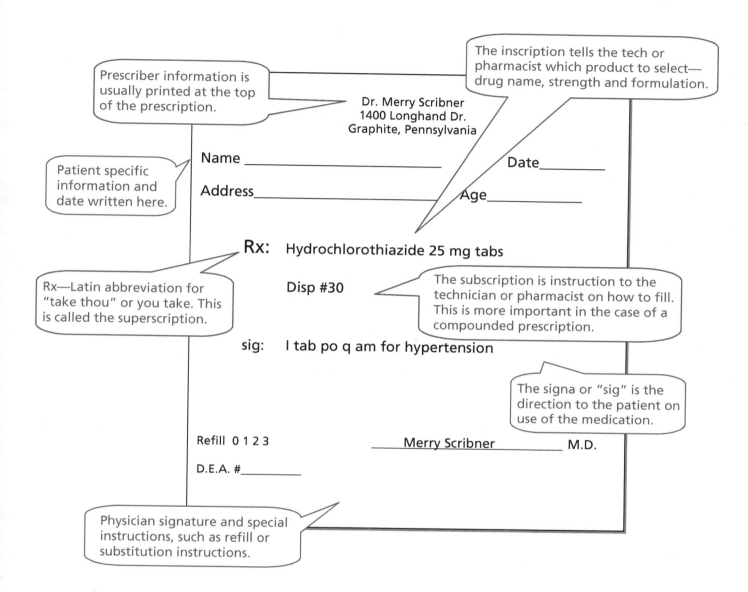

Prescriber information is usually printed at the top of the prescription.

The inscription tells the tech or pharmacist which product to select—drug name, strength and formulation.

Patient specific information and date written here.

Rx—Latin abbreviation for "take thou" or you take. This is called the superscription.

The subscription is instruction to the technician or pharmacist on how to fill. This is more important in the case of a compounded prescription.

The signa or "sig" is the direction to the patient on use of the medication.

Physician signature and special instructions, such as refill or substitution instructions.

Dr. Merry Scribner
1400 Longhand Dr.
Graphite, Pennsylvania

Name _____   Date_____

Address_____ Age_____

Rx: Hydrochlorothiazide 25 mg tabs

Disp #30

sig: I tab po q am for hypertension

Refill 0 1 2 3   ____Merry Scribner____ M.D.

D.E.A. #_____

Appendix B—Conversion Charts

Table B-1. Metric Unit Prefixes, Meanings, and Abbreviations

Prefix	Meaning	Abbreviation
kilo	1000	k
deci	1/10 = 0.1	d
centi	1/100 = 0.01	c
milli	1/1000 = 0.001	m
micro	1/1,000,000 = 0.000001	mc

Table B-2. Common Metric Conversions

Metric units of weight

1 kg	1000 g	1,000,000 mg	1,000,000,000 mcg
	1 g	1000 mg	1,000,000 mcg
		1 mg	1000 mcg

Metric units of volume

1 L	10 dL	100 cL	1000 mL

Metric units of length

1 km	1000 m	100,000 cm	1,000,000 mm
	1 m	100 cm	1000 mm

Table B-3. Household and Apothecary Measures as Used in Text

Measurements of Volume

1 gallon	4 quarts	8 pints	16 cups	128 f ounces	256 tablesponful (T)	768 tsp
	1 quart	2 pints	4 cups	32 f ounces	64 T	192 tsp
		1 pint	2 cups	16 f ounces	32 T	96 tsp
			1 cup	8 f ounces	16 T	32 tsp
				1 f ounce	2 T	6 tsp
					1 T	3 tsp

Measurements of Weight

1 pound	16 ounces

Table B-4. Common Metric, Household, and Apothecary Conversion Factors

Metric Measurement	Household Measurement	Apothecary Measurement
0.065 g (65 mg)		1 grain (gr)
1 g		15.4 grains
28.4 g	1 ounce (oz)	
0.454 kg (454 g)	1 pound (lb)	
1 kg	2.2 lb	
1 L	1.04 quart	
960 mL	1 quart	
480 mL	1 pint	
240 mL	1 cup (8 f oz)	
30 mL	1 f oz	8 fluid drams
15 mL	1 tablespoonful (T)	
5 mL	1 teaspoonful (tsp)	
4 mL		1 fluid dram = 60 minims

Appendix C—Latin Prescription Abbreviations and Medical Terminology

Table C-1. Frequently Used Prescription Abbreviations and Medical Terminology

Abbreviation	Latin	Meaning	Abbreviation	Latin	Meaning
Dosage Forms and Routes of Administration					
cap		capsule	a.d	auris dextro	right ear
gtt(s)	gutta(e)	drop(s)	a.s.	auris sinistro	left ear
liq	liquor	solution or liquid	a.u.	auris utro	both ears
lot.		lotion	bucc	buccal	in the cheek
supp.		suppository	IM		intramuscular
syr.		syrup	inj		injection
sol.		solution	IV		intravenous
susp.		suspension	IVP		IV push
tab		tablet	IVPB		IV piggyback
tr, tinc.		tincture	o.d.	oculo dextro	right eye
			o.s.	oculo sinistro	left eye
			o.u.	oculo utro	both eyes
			p.o.	per os	by mouth
			p.r.		per rectum
			sc or sq		subcutaneous
			Top.		topical
Frequency					
a.c.	ante cibum	before meals	p.m.	postmeridian	afternoon
ad. lib.	ad libitum	as desired	p.r.n.	pro re nata	as needed
a.m.	antemeridian	morning	q	quaque	every
b.i.d.	bis in die	twice a day	q.d.	quaque die	daily
h.s.		at bedtime	q.i.d.	quater in die	four times a day
h		hour	q4h		every 4 hours*
min.		minute	q.o.d.		every other day
noct.	nocte	night	stat		immediately
p.c.	post cibum	after meals	t.i.d	ter in die	three times a day
Other Common Abbreviations					
a	ante	before	NKA		no known allergies
asap		as soon as possible	NPO		nothing by mouth
BM		Bowel movement	NS		normal saline
BP		blood pressure	n/v		nausea/vomiting
DC or d/c		discontinue	p	post	after
dx		diagnosis	SOB		shortness of breath
HA		headache	URI		upper respiratory infection
L or R		left or right	UTI		urinary tract infection
M.R.		may repeat			

*Any number can be used here, i.e., q12h means every 12 hours.

Table C-2. Common Abbreviations Used in Compounding and Their Meanings

Abbreviation	Latin/Early Meaning	Common Usage
aa	ana	of each
ad	ad	up to
aq	aqua	aqueous, water
disp.		dispense
comp.		compound
d.t.d.	dentur tales doses	dispense such doses
mist.	mistura	mix
non rep.	non repetatur	do not repeat; no refills
pulv.	pulvis, pulveris	powder
q.s.	quantum sufficiat	a sufficient quantity
sol.	solutio	solution
ss	semis	one half
ung	unguentum	ointment
u.d. or ut. dict.	ut dictum	as directed

Glossary

Accuracy—The closeness of a measurement to its true value.

Active Ingredient—An active ingredient is the substance in a drug that is biologically active.

Addend—A number that is added to another number.

Adverse Drug Event—Harm resulting from the proper or improper use of a medication in healthcare.

Aliquot—A portion or part of a whole, where most often, the aliquot divides into the whole with no remainder.

Alligation—A practical method used to solve compounding problems where a new strength is made from two different strengths of the same product.

Alligation Alternate—An approach used to solve a different type of strength calculation problem. The alligation alternate method is used to calculate how much of each of two strength products should be combined to create a new product of intermediate specified strength.

Alligation Medial—The process used to find the strength of a product when known amounts of a given concentration are combined. In this process, the amount of drug in the ingredients is determined, and the measured volume or weight of the ingredients is totaled. These sums are then written as a ratio and the new percent strength is calculated.

Annual Depreciation—The loss in value of a long-term asset divided by the estimated life of the asset.

Apothecary—A member of the healing arts who was the predecessor of today's pharmacists.

Average Inventory Value—Sum of inventory values divided by number of inventories.

Average Wholesale Price—A term referring to the average price at which wholesalers sell prescription drugs to pharmacies.

Avoirdupois System—The system of weights and measures historically used in the U.S. and Great Britain.

Body Surface Area—The measured or calculated surface area of the human body, expressed in meters squared.

Calibrated—Marked with measurement lines.

Celsius—A temperature scale in which 0° corresponds to the freezing point of water and 100° corresponds to the boiling point of water.

Centigrade—Another name for the celsius temperature scale.

Compound—Preparation of a product from pharmaceutical-grade ingredients to meet the needs of the patient.

Concentrate—An increased strength of a pharmaceutical preparation used in compounding.

Controlled Substance—A prescription medication identified as having potential for abuse or addiction.

Conversion Factor—A ratio whose value is 1, used to convert between units or systems of measure.

Decimal Fraction—A fraction whose denominator is a power of ten.

Delayed-Release—A dosage form that releases medication at a later time or over an extended period of time.

Denominator—The part of a fraction that is below the fraction bar; also the divisor of a division problem.

Density—The mass of a substance per unit of volume it occupies, reported as g/mL.

Difference—The answer to a subtraction problem.

Diluent—An inert substance used to dilute.

Dilution—The process of making a pharmaceutical preparation less concentrated.

Dimensional Analysis—A method for problem solving that uses conversion factors expressed as fractions and arranged so that any dimensional unit appearing in both numerator and denominator of any of the fractions is canceled until only the desired units remain.

Discount—A reduction from the full or standard amount of a price.

Discount Rate—The percentage by which the price of an item is discounted.

Dividend—A number that is to be divided by a divisor.

Divisor—A number by which another number is to be divided.

Dose—A specified quantity of a therapeutic agent, such as a drug or medicine, prescribed to be taken at one time or at stated intervals.

Dosing Regimen—The expected amount of medication prescribed per time unit and duration of dosing.

Drug Interactions—The alteration of activity, metabolism, or excretion of one drug by another.

Electrolytes—A chemical compound that can conduct electrical current.

Equation—A mathematical statement of equality.

Extemporaneous Compounding—The production of a medication that is not commercially available, in an appropriate dosage form and quantity, from pharmaceutical ingredients.

Factor—That which is multiplied.

Fahrenheit—A temperature scale in which 32° corresponds to the freezing point of water and 212° corresponds to the boiling point of water.

Fraction—A number usually expressed in the form a/b.

Gram—Standard unit of mass in the metric system.

Gross Profit—A business' revenue minus its cost of goods sold.

Improper Fraction—A fraction in which the numerator is greater than the denominator.

Inactive Ingredient—Substances in medication that are not intended to treat symptoms or a health condition.

Infusion—The slow continuous introduction of a solution, especially into a vein.

Integer—Mathematical term to define the set of whole numbers both positive and negative, as well as 0.

International Unit—An internationally agreed upon amount of a substance, based on its biological activity.

Inventory—A complete list of items such as property, goods in stock, or the contents of a building.

Inventory Value—The value of goods held.

Leading Zero—A zero to the left of the decimal point, used in health care to prevent misinterpretation of drug strengths less than one.

Liter—Standard unit of volume in the metric system.

Long-Term Asset—Asset whose value is realized over a period of time.

Markup—The amount added to the cost of goods to cover overhead and profit.

Meter—The standard unit of length in the metric system.

Metric System—The decimal measuring system based on the meter, liter, and gram as units of length, capacity, and weight or mass.

Military Time—A time keeping system based on a 24-hour clock.

Millimole—One thousandth of a mole.

Minimum Weighable Quantity—The smallest amount that can be weighed on a balance with an acceptable error rate.

Mixed Number—A number that consists of a whole number and a fraction.

Mole—One mole of a substance is equal to its atomic or molecular weight in grams and contains 6.022×10^{23} (Avogadro's number) of particles.

Molecular Weight—The average weight of a molecule of a substance, expressed by a number equal to the sum of the atomic weights of all atoms in the molecule.

Net Profit—Amount of money earned after all expenses, including overhead, employee salaries, manufacturing costs, and advertising costs, have been paid.

Number—A number is a label for counting or measuring objects or members of a set.

Numeral—A written symbol used to represent a number.

Numerator—The portion of a fraction above the fraction line.

Outpatient—A patient whose illness is cared for at home.

Over-The-Counter Medication—A medication sold without a prescription for self-use.

Percent—A ratio, represented as parts per 100 parts.

Percent Strength—The concentration of an active ingredient or drug, represented as a percent, in a formulation or mixture.

Place Value—A system of notation where the position of a numeral with respect to a decimal point determines its value.

Precision—The ability of a measurement to be consistently reproduced.

Prescription—A written or electronic order from a physician or other prescriber to the pharmacist, with directions for preparing a medication or providing a device, to be used by an individual patient.

Prime Number—A number, other than 1, whose only factors are one and itself.

Product—The answer to a multiplication problem.

Profit—The difference between revenue and expenses.

Proportion—An equation of two equal ratios.

Quotient—The answer to a division problem.

Ratio—The relationship between two quantities.

Ratio Strength—A ratio that describes a medication concentration, written as 1:x, where x is any number.

Receipts—The amount of money received.

Reciprocal—The result of interchanging the numerator and denominator of a fraction.

Reconstite—To bring a medication to the liquid state by the addition of water or another diluent.

Revenue—The total of all money received from the sale of a firm's product or service during a given period.

Saline Solution—A solution of sodium chloride and distilled water.

Set—A set is a collection of similar, distinct objects.

Short-Term Asset—Asset whose value is realized in a short period of time.

Signa, Sig—Part of the prescription that provides directions to the patient on how to use the medication.

Solute—The substance dissolved in a solution.

Solution—A liquid preparation of one or more substances dissolved in a solvent.

Solvent—The liquid in which a solute is dissolved to form a solution.

Specific Gravity—The relative density of a substance as compared to the density of water under the same conditions.

Sterile—The absence of contaminating microorganisms or infectious particles.

Strength—Labeled potency of a tablet, capsule, or other drug product.

Sum—The answer to an addition problem.

Third Party Payer—A company, organization, insurer, or government agency which makes payment for health care services received by a patient.

Total—The answer to an addition problem.

Trailing Zero—A zero in the decimal representation of a number, after which no other digits follow.

Turnover Rate—Measures the number of times a company sells its inventory during the year.

Unit-Dose System—A system of drug dispensing where a 24-hour supply of medication is dispensed in ready-to-use, single dose packages.

Valence—The capacity of an element to combine with other elements, compared with that of one hydrogen atom.

Variable—The letter or symbol used to represent an unknown quantity.

Answers

Answers to odd-numbered problems are included in this Appendix. All answers are available to instructors at www.ASHP.org/techcalculations.

Chapter 1

1. Use the appendix to answer the following questions about prescriptions and drug orders:
   a. What is a "sig"?

      Directions to the patient on how to use the prescription
   b. What does "Rx" mean?

      Recipare or you take; directions to the pharmacist
   c. Where is information about the prescriber usually found?

      Printed at the top of an outpatient prescription

3. Where are the learning objectives for each chapter located?

   At the beginning of the chapter

5. Use the Internet to find the body surface area of a 5 year-old boy who is 45 inches tall and weighs 40 pounds.

   BSA = 0.76 m²

7. Why do you think it is important to know what a medication is used for before you fill a prescription with it? Write a sentence or two to explain.

   When a technician knows what a drug is used for it helps prevent medication errors. For example, if you only know Viagra® from ads for erectile dysfunction, you would likely question its use in a woman or in an infant. However, if you know a little more, you might be aware that it is a strong vasodilator that is useful in pulmonary hypertension and Raynaud's syndrome.

9. Use the Internet to find a case report of a serious dosing or calculation error. Write up a paragraph on the error and include the following:
   a. What was the cause of the error?
   b. What was the age of the person injured?
   c. Were there procedures or practices that contributed to the error?
   d. How might it have been prevented?

Chapter 2

In pharmacy, Roman numerals are most likely to be encountered when reading a prescription. Convert the following pharmacy-related examples as directed in the problem. Refer to Appendix A (Parts of a Prescription), and Appendix C (Frequently Used Prescription Abbreviations and Medical Terminology), for more information.

1. Convert these Roman numeral volumes to Arabic numerals:
   a. iv fluid ounces

      4 fluid ounces
   b. viii oz

      8 ounces
   c. XII oz

      12 ounces

3. On a prescription, some prescribers write the number of tablets or capsules to be dispensed as Roman numerals. Write the following Arabic numerals as Roman numerals.

  a. 120 tablets

    CXX tablets

  b. 36 capsules

    XXXVI capsules

  c. 24 tabs

    XXIV tabs

5. Write these Roman numeral prescription quantities as Arabic numerals. The abbreviation "disp" means dispense.

  a. Disp # XLV

    Disp #45

  b. Disp xxviii tablets

    Disp 28 tablets

  c. Disp xvi oz

    Disp 16 oz

Answer the following problems about place value:

7. Write the place value names for each digit in the following whole numbers:

  a. 4

    4; units

  b. 55

    55; tens, units

  c. 675

    675; hundreds, tens, units

  d. 12,463

    12,463; ten thousands, thousands, hundreds, tens, units

Round as directed in the problem.

9. Round the following to the nearest 0.5 mL:

  a. 122.9 mL

    123 mL

  b. 1.4 mL

    1.5 mL

  c. 0.72 mL

    0.5 mL

  d. 17.6 mL

    17.5 mL

11. René Norris needs to measure 3.5 mL of Augmentin® 600 for her toddler Joe's ear infection. She has a 5-mL oral syringe, marked in 0.2-mL increments. Can she accurately measure 3.5 mL in the 5-mL syringe?

  Yes, she can draw the Augmentin® suspension up to half-way between the 3.4-mL line and the 3.6-mL line.

13. Patsy Pitts, the pharmacy technician at Save Rite Pharmacy, receives a prescription as follows:

> Promethazine with Codeine
> Disp: viii fl oz

She sees a 16-fluid ounce bottle that appears to be about half full on the shelf. How many ounces of promethazine with codeine will be left after the prescription is filled?

If she dispenses 8 ounces, as ordered, there will be no promethazine with codeine left after filling the prescription. Half of a 16-ounce bottle is 8 ounces.

15. Jenny Jones, C.Ph.T., prepares discharge medications for patients going home from the hospital's surgery center. She receives a discharge prescription with the following Rx:

> Vicodin tablets
> Disp # XLVIII

She has only one bottle of 100 tablets left and has another prescription for 24 tablets. If she dispenses the Vicodin as ordered here, will she have enough left to fill the second prescription?

XLVII = 48

100 tablets – 48 tablets = 52 tablets

She will have enough to fill both prescriptions.

In the following examples there are problems in the way these prescriptions or drug orders are written. List the errors and explain why they are dangerous.

16, 17, 18. There are three examples of error-causing practices in the way the prescription below is written. Based on what you learned in this chapter, identify the problems and explain why they could be dangerous to the patient.

Beatrice Heinz, M.D.
1200 Du LacPlace
Lakeside, Minn

Name: Anne DeLong

Address: 1248 Saint Cloud Drive, Lakeside

Date: 1/1/12

Rx: Levothyroxine 125.0
Disp: xxxx

Sig: One tablet P.O. daily

Refills: 0 1 2 3

Beatrice Heinz _____ M.D.

16, 17, 18. The prescription includes no units with the levothyroxine, which can lead to dose confusion. In addition, a trailing zero is included after 125. This creates opportunity for error, especially if the decimal point is inconspicuous. The Roman numeral XXXX is an incorrectly written Roman numeral. Did the physician intend to write 30, or intend for the patient to receive 40 tablets (XL)? This would require a telephone call for clarification before filling the prescription.

19, 20. The pharmacy department received the following drug order. Find the two problem-prone writing practices in this order and explain why they are dangerous.

> Morphine Sulfate 2 IV Q 2 hours prn pain. If patient becomes overly sedated give Narcan .4 mg SC q 15 minutes prn excess sedation, up to 3 doses.

19, 20. Units are not included in the morphine order and may cause confusion. Does the prescriber intend for the patient to receive 2 mg or 2 mL? In addition, the Narcan® order requires a leading zero. Without it the dose could be interpreted as 4 mg.

Chapter 3

1. **Find the sum.**
   a. $3 + 9 = 12$
   b. $127 + 13 = 140$
   c. On Monday, Bill the pharmacist sees 19 customers for prescription consultations and pharmacist Don sees 18 customers for consultations. Altogether, how many customers were seen for consultations on Monday?
      $19 + 18 = 37$

3. **Find the product.**
   a. $8 \times 7 = 56$
   b. $3 \times 4 \times 14 = 168$
   c. Dr. Dee Kay orders that 2 capsules of Zovirax® 200 mg be administered 5 times daily for 14 days. How many capsules are needed?
      $2 \times 5 \times 14 = 140$

5. **Three hundred vitamin C 250 mg tablets are to be equally distributed among 150 patients.**
   a. How many tablets will each patient receive? Will there be any tablets left over? If so, how many?
      $300 \div 150 = 2$ tablets each, no leftovers
   b. One thousand tablets are to be divided into prescription vials containing 30 tablets each. How many vials are needed? Will there be any tablets left over? If so, how many?
      $1000 \div 30 = 33$ vials with 10 tablets left over

7. **Find the product. Write each product in simplest form.**

   a. $\dfrac{2}{9} \times \dfrac{3}{4} = \dfrac{2 \times 3}{3 \times 3 \times 2 \times 2} = \dfrac{1}{6}$

   b. $\dfrac{9}{28} \times \dfrac{14}{27} = \dfrac{3 \times 3 \times 2 \times 7}{2 \times 2 \times 7 \times 3 \times 3 \times 3} = \dfrac{1}{6}$

   c. $\dfrac{3}{10} \times \dfrac{5}{6} = \dfrac{3 \times 5}{2 \times 5 \times 2 \times 3} = \dfrac{1}{4}$

9. **Find the quotient. Write each quotient in simplest form.**

   a. $\dfrac{2}{27} \div \dfrac{4}{9} = \dfrac{2}{27} \times \dfrac{9}{4} = \dfrac{2 \times 3 \times 3}{3 \times 3 \times 3 \times 2 \times 2} = \dfrac{1}{6}$

   b. $\dfrac{3}{4}$ of an ounce of hydrocortisone 1% is to be divided into three equal parts. How much will each part contain?

   $\dfrac{3}{4} \div 3 = \dfrac{3}{4} \div \dfrac{3}{1} = \dfrac{3}{4} \times \dfrac{1}{3} = \dfrac{1}{4}$

11. **Find the sum or difference. Write each in simplest form.**

    a. $lcd = 12, \ \dfrac{2}{3} + \dfrac{1}{4} = \dfrac{2}{3} \times \dfrac{4}{4} + \dfrac{1}{4} \times \dfrac{3}{3} = \dfrac{8}{12} + \dfrac{3}{12} = \dfrac{11}{12}$

    b. $lcd = 4, \ \dfrac{3}{4} + \dfrac{1}{8} = \dfrac{3}{4} \times \dfrac{2}{2} + \dfrac{1}{8} = \dfrac{6}{8} + \dfrac{1}{8} = \dfrac{7}{8}$

    c. $lcd = 12, \ \dfrac{2}{3} - \dfrac{1}{12} = \dfrac{2}{3} \times \dfrac{4}{4} - \dfrac{1}{12} = \dfrac{8}{12} - \dfrac{1}{12} = \dfrac{7}{12}$

    d. $lcd = 36, \ \dfrac{2}{9} + \dfrac{5}{12} = \dfrac{2}{9} \times \dfrac{4}{4} + \dfrac{5}{12} \times \dfrac{3}{3} = \dfrac{8}{36} + \dfrac{15}{36} = \dfrac{23}{36}$

    e. $lcd = 45, \ \dfrac{8}{9} - \dfrac{2}{5} = \dfrac{8}{9} \times \dfrac{5}{5} - \dfrac{2}{5} \times \dfrac{9}{9} = \dfrac{40}{45} - \dfrac{18}{45} = \dfrac{22}{45}$

13. **Rewrite the improper fraction as a mixed number.**

    a. $\dfrac{14}{3} = 14 \div 3 = 4R2, \text{ so } \dfrac{14}{3} = 4\dfrac{2}{3}$

    b. $\dfrac{21}{5} = 21 \div 5 = 4R1, \text{ so } \dfrac{21}{5} = 4\dfrac{1}{5}$

    c. $\dfrac{14}{9} = 14 \div 9 = 1R5, \text{ so } \dfrac{14}{9} = 1\dfrac{5}{9}$

15. **Find the quotient.**

    a. $6\dfrac{2}{3} \div \dfrac{5}{3} = \dfrac{20}{3} \div \dfrac{5}{3} = \dfrac{20}{3} \times \dfrac{3}{5} = 4$

    b. 3½ ounces of Robitussin DM® is to be divided into portions that are ¼ ounce each. How many portions will there be?

    $3\dfrac{1}{2} \div \dfrac{1}{4} = \dfrac{7}{2} \div \dfrac{1}{4} = \dfrac{7}{2} \times \dfrac{4}{1} = 14$

c. 2½ tsp of amoxicillin suspension is to be given in two equal doses. How many tsp will there be in each dose?

$$2\frac{1}{2} \div 2 = \frac{5}{2} \div \frac{2}{1} = \frac{5}{2} \times \frac{1}{2} = \frac{5}{4} = 1\frac{1}{4}$$

17. **Rewrite the fraction as a decimal fraction.**

a. $\dfrac{3}{8} = \quad 8\overline{)3.000}^{\,0.375}$

b. $\dfrac{9}{10} = \quad 10\overline{)9.0}^{\,0.9}$

c. $\dfrac{4}{5} = \quad 5\overline{)4.0}^{\,0.8}$

19. **Dr. Gohan N. Sumi directs patient Nora Maki to take one capsule of Augmentin® 250 mg three times a day for 14 days. How many capsules should be dispensed?**

$$\frac{3 \text{ capsules}}{\text{day}} \times 14 \text{ days} = 42$$

21. **Wanda Hu gets three prescriptions filled every month. Although her insurance company provides prescription coverage, she pays a co-pay for each prescription. For her birth control tablets she pays $15.00, for her albuterol inhaler she pays $15.00, but for her Advair® inhaler she pays $65.00 each month. What is the average co-pay Wanda pays?**

$$\frac{\$15.00 + \$15.00 + \$65.00}{3} = \$31.67$$

23. **Nat Faste, the representative from Code Blue Insurance Company, has granted approval for Wright Pharmacy to fill a 90-day supply of Evan Tooly's prescription. He takes two ibuprofen 400-mg tablets three times daily. How many tablets do you need to fill this prescription?**

$$\frac{3 \times 2 \text{ tablets}}{\text{day}} \times 90 \text{ days} = 540 \text{ tablets}$$

25. **The pharmacist asks the pharmacy technician to divide 2000 grams of zinc oxide ointment into several sized jars. He would like the technician to fill ten 60-gram jars, eleven 90-gram jars, and six 30-gram jars.**
    a. What is the total amount of zinc oxide used to fill all the jars?
       10(60 g) + 11(90 g) + 6(30 g) = 600 g + 990 g + 180 g = 1770 g
    b. Write the ratio of the amount in the 60-gram jars over the total amount of zinc oxide ointment used and reduce to the simplest form.
       $$600 \text{ g}/1770 \text{ g} = \frac{60}{177} = \frac{2 \times 2 \times \cancel{3} \times 5}{\cancel{3} \times 59} = 20/59$$
    c. Write the fraction determined in Part b as a decimal.
       20/59 = 0.34 when rounded to two decimal places.

Chapter 4

Choose the most appropriate metric unit of weight, volume, or length for the following problems. Choose from the following options: m, cm, mm, L, mL, g, kg, or mg.

1. Medication directions call for 5 *mL* of cough syrup to be given to a child.

3. Soda is sold in bottles containing 2 *L*.

5. A letter weighs about 20–30 *g*.

7. Directions call for 500 *mg* of vitamin C to be taken daily.

9. Rewrite, using a numeral and the appropriate abbreviation.
   a. One hundred fifty milliliters
      150 mL
   b. Thirty-four micrograms
      34 mcg
   c. Sixty-five liters
      65 L
   d. Three hundred thirty milligrams
      330 mg
   e. Nine hundred fifty-five grams
      955 g
   f. Five kilograms
      5 kg

11. Make the following conversions:
    a. 150 mcg to milligrams
       0.15 mg
    b. 2000 mL to liters
       2 L
    c. 845 kg to grams
       845,000 g
    d. 1.575 g to kilograms
       0.001575 kg
    e. 3000 mg to grams
       3 g
    f. 5000 mg to micrograms
       5,000,000 mcg
    g. 5.35 L to milliliters
       5350 mL
    h. 1775 kg to grams
       1,775,000 g
    i. 350 mcg to grams
       0.00035 g
    j. 14.567 g to milligrams
       14,567 mg

13. **Add 300 mL + 4 L + 1.5 L. Express answer in milliliters and in liters.**
    300 mL = 0.3 L
    0.3 L + 4 L + 1.5 L = 5.8 L
    5.8 L × 1000 mL/L = 5800 mL

15. **Add 455 mg + 365 mcg. Express answer in milligrams and in micrograms.**
    365 mcg = 0.365 mg
    455.365 mg × 1000 mcg/mg = 455,365 mcg

17. **Subtract: 3 g – 3 mg. Express answer in grams and milligrams.**
    3 mg = 0.003 g
    2.997 g × 1000 mg/g = 2997 mg

19. **Subtract: 2.5 L – 1.2 L. Express answer in liters and milliliters.**
    1.3 L × 1000 mL/L = 1300 mL

21. **Choose the appropriate conversion factor to convert milligrams to grams.**
    1 g/1000 mg

23. **Choose the appropriate conversion factor(s) to convert mcg to kg.**
    1 mg/1000 mcg × 1 g/1000 mg × 1 kg/1000 g

25. **Anita DeSmall, Ph.T., receives a prescription for levothyroxine 0.125 mg tablets. She fills the prescription with levothyroxine 125 mcg tablets. Use dimensional analysis to determine if Anita dispensed the correct drug.**
    0.125 mg × 1000 mcg/mg = 125 mcg. This is the correct drug.

Chapter 5

1. **Convert the following to milligrams:**
   a. 5 grain = *325* mg
      5 gr × 65 mg/gr = 325 mg
   b. 1.25 grain = *81* mg
      1.25 gr × 65 mg/gr = 81 mg
   c. 1/150 grain = *0.4* mg
      1/150 gr × 65 mg/gr = 0.4 mg
   d. 10 grain = *650* mg
      10 gr × 65 mg/gr = 650 mg

3. **Convert to the units indicated in the first blank, then use that answer to complete the second conversion in each problem below.**
   a. 15 mL = *½ fl oz* = *3 tsp*
      15 mL = ½ fl oz (30 mL/oz); 15 mL x 1 tsp/5 mL = 3 tsp
   b. 1 pint = *480 mL* = *0.48 L*
      16 oz/pt × 30 mL/oz = 480 mL; 480 mL × 1 L/1000 mL = 0.48 L
   c. ½ pint = *¼ quart* = *0.24 L*
      1 qt/2 pints × ½ pint = ¼ qt; ¼ qt × 960 mL/qt × 1 L/1000 mL = 0.24 L
   d. 0.25 L = *250 mL* = *8.3 fl oz*
      0.25 L × 1000 mL/L = 250 mL; 250 m

5. **Number the following in order from 1–6, smallest to largest volume.**
   Solution: convert each quantity to mL and compare

a. liter =   *1000 mL*   6
b. fl oz =   *30 mL*   3
c. tablespoon = *15 mL*   2
d. mL =   *1 mL*   1
e. pint =   *480 mL*   4
f. quart =   *960 mL*   5

7. **Convert the following as indicated in the problem:**
   a. 1.25 L = *1.3 quart*
      1.25 L × 1000 mL/L × 1 qt/960 mL
   b. 8 fl oz = *240 mL*
      30 mL/fl oz × 8 fl oz = 240 mL
   c. 20 mL = *4 tsp*
      20 mL × 1 tsp/5 mL = 4 tsp
   d. 180 mL = *6 fl oz*
      180 mL × 1 fl oz/30 mL = 6 fl oz

9. **Change the following to milligrams:**
   a. 0.4 lb
      0.4 lb × 454 g/lb × 1000 mg/g = 181,600 mg
   b. 1.1 kg
      1.1 kg × 1000 g/kg × 1000 mg/g = 1,100,000 mg
   c. 8 ounces
      8 oz × 28.4 g/oz × 1000 mg/g = 227,200 mg
   d. 20 grains
      20 gr × 1 g/15.4 gr × 1000 mg/g = 1299 mg

In problems 11–14, match the "drug orders" to the correct metric dosage strengths in the list below. (Note*: some pharmaceutical companies equate 60 mg with 1 grain).

11. **Thyroid extract 2 grains PO daily**
    f

13. **Nitroglycerin 1/200 gr SL tab prn chest pain**
    h

15. **Round the conversion factors found in Table 5-3 and the measurements in the problems to check (estimate) whether the following answers are correct. If you believe the answers given are incorrect, explain how you think the error was made.**

    a. Baby John Doe weighs 4 pounds 6 ounces. Odessa Baddun, the technician, receives a drug order for 0.2 mg/kg indomethacin PO × 1 dose. She calculates the dose as 4 mg indomethacin.
       First convert pounds to kg (rounded): 4 lb × 0.5 kg/lb = 2 kg
       Next, calculate dose: 2 kg × 0.2 mg/kg = 0.4 mg
       Correct or incorrect?
       Incorrect. She made a 10-fold dosing error by losing track of the decimal.

    b. You are filling a prescription for crotamiton lotion to treat the entire Peste family for scabies. After bathing, each family member is to apply lotion to the body. They are to repeat this procedure the next day, then shower to remove the lotion the following day. The pharmacist thinks 30 mL should be adequate for each application for the children and 60 mL for the adults. There are two adults and 4 children. The pharmacist calculates that ½ pint total of the lotion is adequate for both treatments for the whole family.

Calculate amount needed for adults, first. Remember 30 mL = 1 ounce.

2 adults, 2 ounces each for 2 doses: 2 adults × 2 oz × 2 treatments = 8 ounces

4 children, 1 ounce each for 2 doses: 4 children × 1 oz × 2 treatments = 8 ounces

Total needed: 16 oz or 1 pint.

Correct or incorrect?

Incorrect. Total required is 1 pint, not ½ pint.

17. The technician at SuperRx Pharmacy receives a new prescription from Mrs. Moody and checks the electronic patient profile to verify the patient information is complete. Technicians at the pharmacy usually get the weight from the patient in pounds and calculate the weight in kilograms. The record indicates Mrs. Moody weighs 113 pounds, or 249 kg. What is wrong with this information and how do you think the error occurred?

The person that did the calculation multiplied pounds × 2.2 lb/kg instead of dividing. Mrs. Moody actually weighs 51.4 kg.

For problems 18–20, calculate the amount required per the drug orders.

19. The veterinarian ordered furosemide 2 mg/kg twice a day for Les Waters' dog, which has heart failure. Round the weight to the nearest kg.

    a. His dog weighs 45 pounds. How much will the dog receive in one dose?

    45 lb × 1 kg/2.2lb = 20 kg (rounded) × 2 mg/kg = 40 mg

    b. Les' prescription indicates the furosemide solution contains 10 mg/mL. What volume will he measure for one dose?

    40 mg × 1 mL/10 mg = 4 mL

21. A physician orders nitroglycerin 1/150 grain to be placed under the tongue for chest pain. The nitroglycerin is available as 0.4 mg and 0.6 mg. Which is correct for this order? (Note: Pharmaceutical companies that make nitroglycerin assume 60 mg = 1 grain.)

    1/150 gr = 0.007 gr

    65 mg/1 gr = x/0.007 gr

    x = 0.45 mg; the 0.4-mg tablet is the correct choice

23. In 1 week during flu season, the pharmacy where you work received six different prescriptions for Hycodan® cough syrup. These include two prescriptions for 4 fl oz, one prescription for 240 mL, one prescription for 180 mL, one prescription for 120 mL, and one prescription for 6 fl oz.

    a. What is the total number of fl oz of Hycodan® dispensed that week?

    (2 x 4 fl oz) + 6 fl oz = 14 fl oz

    240 mL + 180 mL + 120 mL = 540 mL

    540 mL × 1 oz/30 mL = 18 fl oz

    14fl oz + 18 fl oz = 32 fl oz dispensed

    b. How many mL of Hycodan® were dispensed that week?

    32 fl oz × 30 mL/fl oz = 960 mL

25. Dr. Ole Mann still orders acetaminophen with codeine the old-fashioned way. Using the conversion formula provided in this text, how many milligrams of codeine should be in each tablet of the strengths listed below?
    a. Tylenol with codeine ¼ grain
       ¼ grain × 65 mg/gr = 16.25 mg
    b. Tylenol with codeine ½ grain
       ½ grain × 65 mg/gr = 32.5 mg
    c. Tylenol with codeine 1 grain
       1 grain = 65 mg

Chapter 6

1. Dr. Payne orders penicillin G, 5 million units IVPB to be given to patient Anita Little at 2300 and every 4 hours thereafter throughout the day. At what times on a 12-hour clock should the penicillin IVPB be given?
   2300 is 11:00 PM. Therefore, medication should be given at 11:00 PM, 3:00 AM, 7:00 AM, 11:00 AM, 3:00 PM, and 7:00 PM.

3. The records indicate that patient Leigh King was admitted to the hospital at 1600. What time is this on a 12-hour clock?
   1600 – 1200 = 4:00 PM

5. Dr. Lance Boyle orders that patient Ann Teac be given furosemide 20 mg PO at 2400 and every 6 hours thereafter for 24 hours. At what military times should the furosemide be given?
   2400 is midnight (first dose), then 0600 (6:00 AM), 1200 (noon), 1800 (6:00 PM), and last dose at 2400 (midnight).

7. Normal body temperature, measured rectally, is 37.6°C. What is this in Fahrenheit degrees?
   °F = (1.8)°C + 32 = 37.6(1.8) + 32 = 99.7°F

9. Water droplets in clouds are often super cooled, that is they remain liquid at temperatures below the usual freezing point. A cloud droplet will freeze as soon as its temperature drops below –40°C. What is this in degrees Fahrenheit?
   °F = –40(1.8) + 32 = –40°F

11. Sodium bicarbonate should be stored between 15°C and 30°C. What are these temperatures in degrees Fahrenheit?
    °F = 15(1.8) + 32 = 59° F; °F = 30(1.8) + 32 = 86° F. Between 59°F and 86°F

13. Diltiazem should be stored at 77°F, but will tolerate temperatures between 59°F and 86°F for brief periods of transport. What are these temperatures in degrees centigrade?
    °C = (59 – 32)/1.8 = (45)/1.8 = 15°C; °C = (86 – 32)/1.8 = 30°C. Between 15°C and 30°C.

15. Some laboratory specimens must be stored in a freezer in which the temperature ranges from –32°C to –26°C. What are these temperatures in Fahrenheit?
    ° F = –32(1.8) + 32 = –26° F; ° F = –26(1.8) + 32 = –15°F. Between –26°F and –15°F when rounded.

17. On January 16, 2009, the temperature at Big Black River in Maine was −50°F. What is this temperature in centigrade?

°C = (−50 − 32)/1.8 = −46°C

19. Before it is opened, injectable insulin should be stored at 0˚C to 8˚C. Should it be stored in the refrigerator, freezer, or at room temperature?

F = 1.8(0) + 32 = 32°F; °F = 1.8(8) + 32 = 46°F. Refrigerator temperatures range from 32°F − 46°F; therefore, refrigerate the medication.

Chapter 7

1. List eight pieces of information required on a prescription.

Patient name and address
Name, form, and strength of the medication
Quantity of the medication to dispense
Directions to the patient (route of administration, frequency of administration)
Date written
Prescriber name and address
Prescriber signature
Prescriber classification

3. Write the meaning of the following routes of administration:
   a. p.o.
      by mouth
   b. IVP
      IV push
   c. IM
      intramuscular
   d. top
      topical

5. Interpret the following drug orders as a nurse might read them and write out your interpretation.
   a. Zosyn 2.25 g IVPB Q8H
      Give Zosyn 2.25 g by intravenous piggyback every 8 hours.
   b. Morphine sulfate 5 mg sc q3H prn moderate pain or S.O.B.
      Give morphine sulfate 5 mg by subcutaneous injection every 3 hours if needed for moderate pain or shortness of breath.
   c. NS 1000 mL IV to run at 125 mL/hr
      Infuse 1000 mL normal saline intravenously at a rate of 125 mL per hour.
   d. Naloxone 0.4 mg IVP stat and q 15–30 min prn respiratory depression
      Give naloxone 0.4 mg by intravenous push immediately and repeat every 15 to 30 minutes if needed for respiratory depression.

7. Check the following DEA numbers to see if they meet the test for validity. Indicate why you think they could be valid or are invalid.
   a. Wilma Ruth, MD, DEA Registration # A.R. 1234563
      1. 1 + 3 + 5 = 9   2. 2 + 4 + 6 = 12   3. 2 × 12 =24   4. 24 + 9 = 33
      Could be valid

b. Daniel Bones, MD, DEA. Registration # B.D. 2754388
   Could be valid

c. Rebecca Darling, DVM, DEA Registration # B.D 5704386
   Could be valid

9. **Write the abbreviations that correspond to the following words or phrases.**
   a. capsule
      cap
   b. suspension
      susp
   c. after meals
      pc
   d. twice a day
      BID
   e. as directed
      UD
   f. no known allergies
      NKA

11. **Lantus® Insulin expires 28 days after the vial is opened. If the patient in problem 10 uses his insulin as ordered, how much will be left in the vial after 28 days?**
    0.15 mL/day × 28 days = 4.2 mL used. 10 mL – 4.2 mL = 5.8 mL remaining.

13. **List four routes of administration by which medication may be administered.**
    PO (by mouth), IV (intravenous), SC (subcutaneous injection), IM (intramuscular injection), TOP (topical), SL (sublingual), and others.

15. **Write out the directions listed below completely, as you would type them on a prescription label.**
    a. ii gtts o.s. qid while awake
       Instill two (2) drops in the left eye four times a day, while awake.
    b. 15 mL p.o. q4h prn cough or congestion
       Take one tablespoonful (15 mL) by mouth every 4 hours if needed for cough or congestion.
    c. i tab sl q 5 min × 3 prn chest pain
       Place one tablet under the tongue if needed for chest pain. May repeat every five (5) minutes for 3 doses if chest pain persists.
    d. caps ii p.o. B.I.D for blood pressure
       Take two (2) capsules by mouth twice a day for blood pressure.

17. **Calculate the number of tablets needed to fill the following prescription:**
    Rx: Azithromycin 250 mg tablets
    Disp: 5 day supply
    Sig: tabs ii now, then i tab daily
    2 (now) + (1 tab/day × 4 days) = 6 tablets

19. **You receive the following prescription for amoxicillin suspension for a child with an acute middle ear infection:**
    Amoxicillin susp. 400 mg/5 mL
    320 mg (4 mL) Q8H × 7 days

Amoxicillin 400 mg/5 mL for suspension is available in 50 mL, 75 mL, and 100 mL bottles. Which size will you dispense?

4 mL/dose × 3 doses/day = 12 mL/day

12 mL/day × 7 days = 84 mL; therefore the 100-mL bottle is necessary

21. **For each of the sigs given below, state how many doses the patient will receive in 1 day.**

a. Q2h

24 h/day × 1 dose/2 h = 12 doses/day

b. TID

3 doses/day

c. Q8h

24 h/day × 1 dose/8 h = 3 doses/day

23. **The pharmacist receives the following prescription for compounding:**

Drug A	60 mL
Drug B	500 mg
Alcohol 70%	60 mL
Lotion C qs ad	200 mL

a. What does qs ad mean?

Quantity sufficient to make

b. The pharmacy has a 6-ounce bottle of lotion C on the shelf. Will that be enough to compound the prescription?

Drug A + alcohol = 120 mL

200 mL – 120 mL = 80 mL maximum. 6 ounces is enough.

25. **For each of the past 4 weeks, the usage of Vicodin® tablets from the automated dispensing cabinet you fill is as follows:**

Week 1: 86 tablets   Week 3: 93 tablets

Week 2: 120 tablets   Week 4: 112 tablets

a. How many Vicodin® tablets are used in an average week?

103 (rounded)

b. The current tablet count in the drawer is 7 tablets and the maximum for the drawer is 125 tablets. How many tablets should you add to reach the maximum?

125 – 7 = 118 tablets

Chapter 8

Solve the following equations.

1. $\dfrac{1}{10}x = 25$

$\dfrac{1}{10}x = 25$

$10 \times \dfrac{1}{10}x = 10 \times 25$

$x = 250$

3. $100x = 50$

$100x = 50$

$$\frac{100x}{100} = \frac{50}{100}$$

$$x = \frac{1}{2}$$

5. $30x + 15 = 345$

$30x + 15 = 345$

$30x + 15 - 15 = 345 - 15$

$30x = 330$

$$\frac{30x}{30} = \frac{330}{30}$$

$x = 11$

Identify the unknown (define the variable) in the following situations.

7. Ritalin® is available in 20-mg scored tablets. How many tablets should be given per dose if the dose is 30 mg?

   Let x = the number of tablets that should be given in one dose.

9. A prescription calls for 40 mg of furosemide to be given four times daily. How many milligrams of furosemide will be taken daily?

   Let x = the number of milligrams of furosemide taken daily.

Identify the unknown (define the variable) in the following situations. Make an estimate of the answer.

11. A prescription for risperidone 1 mg calls for 1 tablet three times daily for one day, then two tablets twice a day for one day, then three tablets twice a day for seven days. How many tablets are needed to fill the prescription?

    Let x = the number of tablets needed to fill the prescription. Estimate 45 to 50 (3tabs BID = 6/day for 7 days plus extras).

13. A prescription calls for one tablet to be taken four times a day. Ninety tablets are dispensed. How many days should this prescription last?

    Let x = the number of days the prescription should last. Estimate 20–25 days (round 90 to 100 and divide by 4).

15. Seventy-two percent of a 500-mL solution is water. How many milliliters of the solution is water?

    Let x = the number of milliliters of water. Estimate 375 mL (75% or ¾ of 500 mL).

Identify the unknown (define the variable) in the following situations. Make an estimate of the answer. Translate the situation to an equation. Solve the equation and check solution for reasonableness with your original estimate.

17. A pharmacist had 2 g of Drug C. He used it to prepare the following:

    8 capsules each containing 0.0325 g

    12 capsules each containing 0.015 g

    18 capsules each containing 0.0008 g

    How many grams of Drug C were left after he prepared the capsules?
    Let x = number of grams of Drug C that are left.
    x = 2 − 8(0.0325) − 8(0.015) − 12(0.0008)
    x = 1.6104

19. A prescription written for penicillin VK 250-mg tablets instructs that one tablet be taken every 6 hours.
    a. How many tablets should the patient take each day?
       Let x = number of tablets the patient should take each day.

       $x = \dfrac{1 \; tablet}{6 \; hours} \times 24 \; hours$

       x = 4 tablets

    b. If the pharmacist dispenses 28 tablets, how long should the prescription last?
       Let x = number of days the prescription will last.

       $x = \dfrac{28 \; tablets}{4 \; tablets/day}$

       x = 7 days

21. Zyrtec® is available in scored 10-mg tablets. A patient takes 5 mg daily for 30 days. How many tablets are needed?
    Let x = number of 10-mg Zyrtec® tablets

    $x = \dfrac{5 \; mg}{day} \times \dfrac{\frac{1}{2} \; tablet}{5 \; mg} \times 30 \; day = 15 \; tablets$

23. On Monday, Ivan Aik filled his prescription for 75 Vicodin® 500-mg tablets. He takes them as needed for pain, up to eight tablets per day. By Sunday morning (6 days later), 3/5 of the original 75 tablets are left.
    a. How many are left?
    Let x = number of Vicodin® tablets that are left.

    $x = \dfrac{3}{5} \, (75)$

    x = 45
    There are 45 tablets left
    b. How many Vicodin® tablets did Ivan take?
       Let y = the number of tablets Ivan took
       y = 75 − 45
       y = 30
       Ivan took 30 Vicodin® tablets.

   c. If Ivan took the same number of tablets each day, did he take more than eight tablets per day?

     Let D = number of tablets taken per day

     D = 30 tablets/6 days

     D = 5 tablets/day

     No, Ivan did not take more than eight tablets per day.

25. Karl Kardyo takes warfarin 5 mg once a day for three months (90 days). How many milligrams of warfarin does Karl take in 3 months?

   Let x = number of mg of warfarin taken in 3 months

   x = (5 mg/day)(90 days)

   x = 450 mg

   Karl takes 450 mg of warfarin in 3 months.

Chapter 9

1. Write the following statements as ratios:

   a. Many potato salad recipes call for 6 cups of peeled and chopped potatoes for 8 servings of potato salad.

     6 c potatoes/8 servings

   b. Jennifer drives 475 miles on 10.5 gallons of gas in her new Prius.

     475 miles/10.5 gal

   c. Mylanta suspension costs $6.99 for 12 oz.

     $6.99/12oz

   d. There are 900 calories in a double cheeseburger.

     900cal/1 double cheeseburger

3. Write the following ratios as fractions:

   a. 3:4

     3/4

   b. 1:10

     1/10

   c. 9:1000

     9/1000

   d. 2:3

     2/3

5. **On the following drug labels, find the drug strength per mL:**

a.

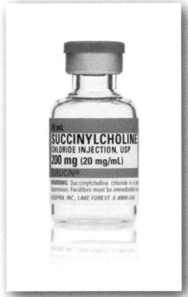

Source: Reprinted with permission of Hospira, Inc.

20 mg/mL

b.

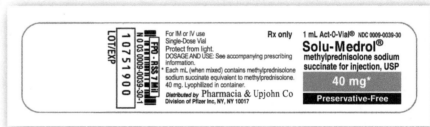

Source: Reprinted with permission of Pfizer Inc.

40 mg/mL

7. **A vial of furosemide for injection contains 40 mg/4 mL. What volume of furosemide for injection contains 10 mg?**

   40 mg/4 mL = 10 mg/x   x = 1 mL

9. **Epinephrine is available in a 1:1000 solution and a 1:10,000 solution.**

   a. Which product contains more epinephrine per mL?

   1:1000 means 1 gram/1000 mL and 1:10,000 means 1 g/10,000 mL, so 1:1000 contains more.

   b. How many mg of epinephrine are in 10 mL of a 1:10,000 solution?

   1000 mg/10,000 mL = x/10 mL

   x = 1 mg

11. The ABC pharmacy in the pediatrics clinic carries erythromycin ethyl succinate suspension in a concentration of 400 mg/5 mL. Dr. Darlene Bebe ordered a dose of 300 mg Q6 hours and wants a 10-day supply for her patient.

   a. What volume of the suspension contains 300 mg erythromycin ethyl succinate?

   400 mg/5 mL = 300 mg/x

   x = 3.75 mL

   b. Should the pharmacy dispense the 100-mL bottle or the 200-mL bottle to provide enough for 10 days?

   24 h/d × 1 dose/6 hours = 4 doses/day

   3.75 mL/dose × 4 doses/day = 15 mL/day or 150 mL in 10 days

   dispense the 200-mL bottle

13. Phenytoin oral suspension contains 125 mg of the drug in 5 mL. The physician orders 250 mg to be given every 12 hours.

   a. What volume of the suspension will the patient receive per dose?

   125 mg/5 mL = 250 mg/x

   x = 10 mL

   b. When taken according to the directions, how many mL will the patient receive in a day?

   10 mL/dose × 2 doses/day = 20 mL/day

   c. How long will an 8-fl oz bottle last?

   240 mL/bottle × 1 day/20 mL = 12 days/bottle

15. Solve the following proportion equations:

   a. 1:10,000 :: 5:*x*

   Read 1 is to 10,000 as 5 is to x. Equation may be rewritten 1/10,000 = 5/x, or solved as follows: 1(x) = 5(10,000)

   x = 50,000

   b. 1 gram/10 mL = *x*/350 mL

   x(10 mL) = 1 g(350 mL)

   x = 35 g

   c. 500 mcg/2 mL = 750 mcg/*x*

   x (500 mcg) = 750 mcg (2 mL)

   x = 3 mL

   d. 3:18 :: *x*:162

   3(162) = 18(x)

   x = 27

17. A 20-mL multidose vial of vaccine costs $475. One dose of vaccine is 0.5 mL.

   a. How many people can be vaccinated with one vial?

   20 mL/0.5 mL/dose = 40 doses; therefore, 40 people can be vaccinated

   b. What is the cost per dose of vaccine?

   $475/40 doses = $11.88/dose

19. You are planning a pizza party for the pharmacy department. On average, each person usually eats three slices of pizza, and a large pie contains 12 slices. There are 17 pharmacists and technicians coming. How many large pizzas should you order to make sure there is enough for 3 slices each?

   3 slices/person × 17 persons = 51 slices of pizza needed

   1 pizza/12 slices × 51 slices needed = 4.25 pizzas, or 5 pizzas to feed everyone

21. Deanna, the dietician, is talking to Betty Baker, recently diagnosed with diabetes, about her diet. Betty loves to make apple pies. Deanna says the calories in a 9-inch apple pie come from 260 g carbohydrates (from apples, sugar, and flour) and 110 g fat. The entire pie contains 2030 calories.

    a. If the pie is divided in 8 equal pieces, how many calories are in 3 pieces?

    2030 cal/8 pieces = x/3 pieces

    x = 761.25 cal

    b. There are 1040 calories provided by the 260 g of carbohydrates in the whole pie. How many calories does 1 gram of carbohydrate provide?

    1040 cals/260 g carbs = 4 cal/g carbohydrate

    c. If the remaining calories come from 110 grams of fat, how many calories are derived from 1 gram of fat?

    2030 total cal − 1040 cal (from carbs) = 990 cal from fat

    990 cal/110g fat = 9 cal/g fat

23. Our Town Pharmacy is running out of the ingredients for the formulation in Problem 22. The pharmacist asks you to order erythromycin and hydroxypropyl cellulose to make 3-month's supply of the erythromycin 2% gel. She says that the average amount compounded in 1 month is 2.5 liters. The powder is available in 500-g containers and the hydroxypropyl cellulose is available in 1-pound containers. How many containers of each will you order?

    2 grams of each ingredient are needed for each 100 mL

    Number of batches of the 100 mL formulation needed/month: 2500 mL/100 mL = 25 batches/month

    25 batches/mo × 2 g/batch × 3 months = 150 g used in 3 months.

    Therefore, order one container of each.

25. Riley Quick, C.Ph.T., and Nita Gallop, C.Ph.T., have decided to see who is fastest at counting and pouring medication for prescriptions. Nita does the counting and pouring for 43 prescriptions in 3.5 hours. How many prescriptions will Riley need to prepare in his 7.5-hour shift to beat Nita?

    Nita's rate: 43 prescriptions/3.5 hours = 12.3 prescriptions/hr

    Riley must fill more than: 12.3 prescriptions/hr × 7.5 hours = 92.25 prescriptions

    If Riley fills 93 prescriptions or more in 7.5 hours he will beat Nita's rate.

Chapter 10

1. A drug order from the nursing home your pharmacy services reads "venlafaxine 56.25 mg p.o. BID." The pharmacy carries 37.5-mg tablets and 75-mg tablets.

    a. What strength tablets will you use to fill this order and why?

    You will provide 37.5-mg tabs because they require the least amount of tablet splitting, thereby being most safe and convenient for the patient.

    b. How many tablets will the patient take per dose?

    1½ of the 37.5 mg tablets = 56.25 mg

3. Hedda Aiken is an 18-month-old admitted to the pediatric hospital with meningitis. The admitting physician orders Rocephin®, 80 mg/kg/day, in two divided doses. Hedda weighs 19 pounds.

    a. What is Hedda's weight in kg?

    19 lb × 1 kg/2.2 lb = 8.64 kg

b. How many milligrams of Rocephin® will Hedda receive?

8.64 kg × 80 mg/kg = 691 mg (round to 700 mg for accurate measuring)

c. The hospital carries Rocephin® in a ready-to-use formulation that contains 1 gram in 50 mL. What volume will you draw up to fill Hedda's order?

1 g/50 mL = 0.7 g/x

x = 35 mL

5. **You are making IVPB solutions. There are three different orders for gentamicin piggybacks. You have available a 30-mL vial of gentamicin 40 mg/mL.**

a. What volume of gentamicin solution will you draw up in a syringe to make a 60 mg IVPB?

40 mg/1 mL = 60 mg/x

x = 1.5 mL

b. What volume of gentamicin do you need to make a 100-mg piggyback bag?

40 mg/1 mL = 100 mg/x

x = 2.5 mL

c. After making two 60-mg doses, one 100-mg dose, and three 80-mg doses, how much gentamicin will be left in the vial?

40 mg/mL × 30 mL/vial = 1200 mg/vial:

Amount remaining = 1200 mg – amount used

Amount used = 60 mg (2) + 100 mg + 80 mg (3) = 460 mg used

1200 mg – 460 mg = 740 mg remaining

7. **Mrs. Berry is a frequent customer at Small's Pharmacy. Her 7-month-old, 16-pound son has a fever of 103°F. She asks you to double-check her dose calculation, based on the dose of ibuprofen the pharmacist recommended of 10 mg/kg with a maximum of 4 doses/day.**

a. How much ibuprofen should the baby receive per dose?

16 lb × 1 kg/2.2 lb = 7.3 kg

7.3 kg × 10 mg/kg = 73 mg

b. Mrs. Berry chooses ibuprofen children's suspension, which contains 100 mg ibuprofen in 5 mL. What volume of ibuprofen will her son receive per dose in part A?

100 mg/5 mL = 73 mg/x

x = 3.7 mL (rounded)

9. **Convert the following weights to pounds:**

a. *17.7 kg × 2.2 lb/kg = 39 lb*

b. *106 kg × 2.2 lb/kg = 233.2 lb*

c. *65 kg × 2.2 lb/kg = 143 lb*

d. *36 kg × 2.2 lb/kg = 79.2 lb*

11. **How many days will a 10-mL vial of insulin last, when used correctly, for each of the orders above?**

a. *1 day/0.22 mL(10 mL) = 45 days; however, insulin is only good for 28 days after opening*

b. *1 day/0.9 mL x 10 mL = 11 days*

c. *1 day/0.21 mL x 10 mL = 47 days; however, insulin is only good for 28 days after opening*

13. You need to prepare a syringe of heparin containing 22,500 units. The vial of heparin contains 10,000 units per mL. What volume of heparin will you draw up?

10,000 units/1 mL = 22,500 units/x

x = 2.25 mL

15. An oncologist has ordered vinblastine 4 mg/m² to be given every week by slow IV push. The patient weighs 115 pounds and is 62 inches tall. What is the weekly dose (mg) of vinblastine?

Patient's BSA = 1.5 m²

1.51 m² × 4 mg/m² = 6.04 mg or 6.0 mg (rounded) vinblastine/week

17. There is a levothyroxine injection shortage and the hospital has four postoperative patients that need this medication. The pharmacy will draw up a syringe for the patients, but a new single-dose vial must be used each day. The doses are as follows: 125 mcg, 0.175 mg, 100 mcg, and 0.075 mg each day. Each vial contains 0.5 mg levothyroxine.

a. What is the total amount (in milligrams) of levothyroxine used each day?

125 mcg = 0.125 mg, 100 mcg = 0.1 mg

Total mg/day = 0.125 mg + 0.175 mg + 0.1 mg + 0.075 mg = 0.475 mg

b. The hospital has 8 vials left. How long will they last?

8 days

19. A prescriber orders acetaminophen 10-grain suppository for a bedridden hospice patient, whose husband comes in to pick up the medication. The pharmacy carries acetaminophen suppositories in 120-mg, 325-mg, and 650-mg strengths. Which strength should he purchase?

65 mg = 1 grain; therefore, 650 mg = 10 grains

For problems 21–24, refer to the case below:
A physician has ordered Trileptal® suspension 300 mg/5 mL for a boy with a seizure disorder. The child is to receive 10 mg/kg/day initially, in two divided doses, with the dose to be increased gradually over time. The child weighs 44 pounds.

21. What is the child's weight in kg, and how much Trileptal® will he receive initially, per day, and per dose?

44 lb × 1 lb/2.2 kg = 20 kg

20 kg × 10 mg/kg/day = 200 mg/day divided into 2 doses = 100 mg/dose

23. Eventually the child's dose is increased until he is receiving Trileptal® suspension 600 mg BID. What volume will his mother measure to deliver a 600-mg dose of the medication?

300 mg/5 mL = 600 mg/x; x = 10 mL

25. Tracy Tan is a 20-month-old girl with a serious bacterial infection. Her physician orders ceftriaxone 50 mg/kg/day, in two divided doses, to be started immediately. Tracy weighs 21.5 pounds.

a. What is Tracy's weight in kg?

21.5 lb × 1 kg/2.2 lb = 9.8 kg

b. How many mg of ceftriaxone will Tracy receive per day and per dose? Round the daily dose to the nearest 100 mg.

9.8 kg × 50 mg/kg/day = 500 mg/day, 250 mg/dose

Chapter 11

1. **Write the following as percents:**

   a. 0.15

   15 parts per 100 or 15%

   b. 22/100

   22%

   c. 0.63

   63%

   d. 3/4

   0.75 or 75%

   e. 1.1

   110%

   f. 17/24

   0.71 or 71%

3. **From the labels shown, decide whether percentage strengths would be w/w or w/v.**

**HYDROCORTISONE OINTMENT
USP, 1%**

Drug Facts

Active ingredients (in each gram)	Purpose
Hydrocortisone 10 mg.	Anti-itch

Uses · for temporary relieve of itching associated with minor skin irritations and rashes due to: · eczema · insect bites · soaps and detergents · cosmetics · jewelry · seborrheic dermatitis · psoriasis · poisin ivy, oak or sumac · for external genital, feminine and anal itching · other uses of this product should be only under the advice and supervision of a doctor.

Warnings
For external use only
Do not use · in children under 2 years of age · if you have a vaginal discharge · for the treatment of diaper rash

Ask a doctor before use if you have · external genital or feminine itching · external anal itching · bleeding

When using this product · avoid contact with eyes · do not exceed the recommended daily dosage unless directed by a doctor · do not put this product into the rectum by using fingers or any mechanical devices or applicator

Stop use and ask a doctor · if condition worsens, or if symptoms persist for more than 7 days or clear up and occur again within a few days, stop use and do not begin use of any other hydrocortisone product

Keep out of reach of children. If swallowed, get medical help or contact a Poison Control Center right away.

   a. *mg/g = w/w*

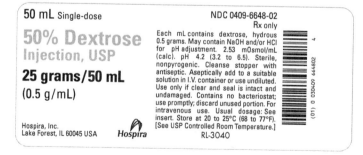

50 mL Single-dose

50% Dextrose
Injection, USP

25 grams/50 mL
(0.5 g/mL)

Hospira, Inc.
Lake Forest, IL 60045 USA

NDC 0409-6648-02
Rx only
Each mL contains dextrose, hydrous 0.5 grams. May contain NaOH and/or HCl for pH adjustment. 2.53 mOsmol/mL (calc). pH 4.2 (3.2 to 6.5). Sterile, nonpyrogenic. Cleanse stopper with antiseptic. Aseptically add to a suitable solution in I.V. container or use undiluted. Use only if clear and seal is intact and undamaged. Contains no bacteriostat; use promptly; discard unused portion. For intravenous use. Usual dosage: See insert. Store at 20 to 25°C (68 to 77°F). [See USP Controlled Room Temperature.]
RL-3040

   Source: Reprinted with permission of Hospira, Inc.

   b. *g/mL = w/v*

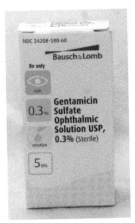

Source: Reprinted with permission of Bausch & Lomb, Inc.

   c. *mg/mL = w/v*

5. Write the following percents as ratios, including appropriate units:

   a. 0.9% (w/v)

     0.9 g/100 mL

   b. 0.75% (v/v)

     0.75 mL/100 mL

   c. 10% (w/w)

     10 g/100 g

7. How much pure ethanol is in 500 mL 70% (v/v) ethanol solution?

   70%(v/v) = 70 mL/100 mL

   70 mL/100 mL = x/500 mL

$$x = \frac{70 \text{ mL (500 mL)}}{100 \text{ mL}} = 350 \text{ mL}$$

9. You are asked to make 240 mL of 3% hydrogen peroxide from the available 6% hydrogen peroxide solution and sterile water for irrigation. How much of each ingredient is needed to make the preparation? (Note: 3% hydrogen peroxide is half as strong as 6%.)

   120 mL of sterile water plus 120 mL of 6% hydrogen peroxide will make 240 mL of 3% hydrogen peroxide.

11. Dexamethasone for injection is available as 4 mg/mL and 10 mg/mL. What are the percent strengths of each product?

   4 mg × 1 g/1000 mg = 0.004 g in each mL or 0.4 g/100 mL = 0.4%

   10 mg × 1 g/1000 mg = 0.01 g; 0.01 g in each mL or 1 g/100 mL = 1%

13. It is a hot summer day in Southern California where you are vacationing, and you hear on the radio that carbon monoxide levels are above the healthy range at 11 PPM. Express this concentration as a percent and as a ratio.

   11 ÷ 1,000,000 = 0.00011% or 11 parts/1,000,000 parts

15. You are to compound one pound of 3% hydrocortisone cream from cream base and hydrocortisone powder.

   a. How much hydrocortisone is contained in one pound of the cream?

   3% = 3 g/100 g; 1 lb = 454 g

   3 g/100 g = x/454 g

   $x = \dfrac{3\ g\ (454\ g)}{100\ g} = 13.62\ g\ hydrocortisone\ in\ 1\ lb\ of\ 3\%\ cream$

   b. How much of the cream base is needed for this product?

   454 g total − 13.62 g hydrocortisone = 440.38 g base

   c. Is this a w/w or w/v problem?

   w/w

17. **Bumetanide for injection contains bumetanide 1 mg/mL. What is the percent strength?**

   1 mg/mL = 100 mg/100 mL or 0.1 g/100 mL = 0.1%

19. **Mometasone cream contains 45 mg mometasone in 45 grams of cream. What percent strength is the cream?**

   45 mg × 1 g/1000 mg = 0.045 g; 0.045 g/45 g = 0.1%

21. **You are making a 1-liter intravenous solution with 250 mL of 50% dextrose and 750 mL of amino acids, electrolytes, and sterile water.**

   a. What is the final concentration of dextrose in the 1-liter bag?

   50% = 50 g/100 mL; 50g/100 mL = x/250 mL

   x = 125 g dextrose. Final solution contains 125 g/1000 mL or 12.5% dextrose

   b. Of the 750 mL added to the dextrose, 500 mL is 7% amino acids solution. What is the final concentration of amino acids in 1 liter?

   7% = 7 g/100 mL; 7 g/100 mL = x/500 mL

   x = 35g amino acid. Final solution contains 35 g/1000 mL or 3.5% amino acid

23. **The local veterinarian would like 10 mL of phenobarbital for injection in a 7.5% solution. You have on hand 65 mg/mL and 130 mg/mL.**

   a. What are the percent strengths of the 65 mg/mL and 130 mg/mL solutions for injection?

   65 mg/1 mL = 6500 mg/100 mL or 6.5%; 130 mg/1 mL = 13,000 mg/100 mL or 13%

   b. How many mL of each strength phenobarbital for injection is needed to make 10 mL of 7.5% solution?

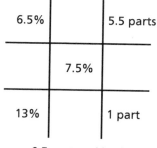

$$\frac{6.5\ parts}{10\ mL} = \frac{5.5\ parts}{x}$$

$$x = 8.46\ mL\ of\ 6.5\%\ phenobarbital\ injection$$

$$\frac{6.5\ parts}{10\ mL} = \frac{1\ part}{y}$$

$$y = 1.54\ mL\ of\ 13\%\ phenobarbital\ solution$$

25. Normal saline solution contains is a 0.9% sodium chloride (NaCl). Other saline solutions are known as ½ normal saline and ¼ normal saline, because they are ½ and ¼ the concentration of normal saline.

   a. What is the percent strength of ½ normal saline?
   0.9% × ½ = 0.45%
   b. What is the percent strength of ¼ normal saline?
   0.9% × ¼ = 0.225%

Chapter 12

1. You work in a compounding pharmacy where the elderly gastroenterologist sends his patients for his special GI upset capsules. Each capsule contains hyoscyamine 0.1 mg, bismuth subsalicylate 500 mg, and famotidine 10 mg. The pharmacist asks you to make 150 capsules. How much of each ingredient will you need?
   Hyoscyamine – 150 × 0.1 mg = 15 mg
   Bismuth subsalicylate – 150 × 500 mg = 75,000 mg = 75 grams
   Famotidine – 150 × 10 mg = 1500 mg = 1.5 grams

3. Advil® Cold and Sinus Caplets each contain ibuprofen 200 mg and pseudoephedrine 30 mg. How much of each ingredient will the manufacturer use to make a bottle of 60 caplets?
   Ibuprofen 60 × 200 mg = 12,000 mg = 12 grams
   Pseudoephedrine 60 × 30 mg = 1800 mg = 1.8 grams

Answer questions 4–6 using the formula for mouthwash, below.
The hospital where you work prepares a mouthwash for patients with stomatitis (mouth sores) called "magic mouthwash" that contains the following:

Hydrocortisone 100 mg/2 mL	2 mL
Nystatin suspension	30 mL
Viscous lidocaine 2%	50 mL
Diphenhydramine elixir 12.5 mg/5 mL q.s a.d	240 mL

5. How much diphenhydramine elixir was necessary for the original formula?
   Total volume – volume of all other ingredients = volume of diphenhydramine
   240 mL – (2 mL + 30 mL + 50 mL) = 158 mL of diphenhydramine

7. The children's hospital where you work dilutes heparin flush 100 units/mL in normal saline for injection to make a special low-dose heparin flush syringe for newborns. The low-dose solution contains 1 unit heparin/mL and each syringe contains 0.5 mL. Your boss asks you to make 50 of these syringes.

    a. How much heparin is contained in 50 of the low-dose heparin flush syringes?

       1 unit/mL × 0.5 mL per syringe × 50 syringes = 25 units in 50 syringes

    b. How much of the heparin 100 units/mL will you use to make the dilute flush solution?

       100 units/mL = 25 units/x

       x = 0.25mL of the heparin 100 units/mL for 50 syringes

    c. How much normal saline for injection will you add to the heparin in Part b to make the dilute heparin flush solution?

       50 syringes × 0.5 mL per syringe = 25 mL total solution

       25 mL – 0.25 mL of the heparin 100 unit/mL needed = 24.75 mL of saline needed.

9. The sensitivity rating of your balance is 6 mg and the acceptable error rate is 3.5%. What is the minimum weighable quantity?

$$\frac{SR \times 100}{\%\ error} = MWQ$$

$$\frac{6\ mg\ (100)}{3.5} = 171\ mg$$

11. In the pediatrics unit of your hospital, a physician orders morphine for a patient who has undergone surgery and is in pain. The morphine is to be drawn up into a 10-mL syringe and administered via a pump that can deliver as little as 0.5 mL/hr. The orders are for morphine 0.25 mg per hour with instruction for the nurse to increase the dose as needed to a maximum of 0.75 mg per hour. The pharmacist tells you to use 10 mg/mL morphine diluted with normal saline to make 10 mL of morphine 0.5 mg/mL.

    a. How much morphine is contained in 10 mL of morphine 0.5 mg/mL?

       0.5 mg/mL = x/10 mL

       x = 5 mg

    b. How much of the morphine 10 mg/mL is needed to make the dilute solution?

       10 mg/1 mL = 5 mg/x

       x = 0.5 mL of the morphine sulfate 10 mg/mL concentration

    c. How much normal saline will be used to make the dilute solution?

       10 mL total – 0.5 mL morphine = 9.5 mL of normal saline

    d. What volume of the dilute solution contains 0.25 mg of morphine?

       0.5 mg/mL = 0.25 mg/x

       x = 0.5 mL

13. An antacid product contains 650 mg calcium carbonate and 500 mg sorbitol in each tablet. Each bottle contains 120 tablets. How much of each ingredient is needed to make 1000 bottles?

   120 tablets/bottle × 650 mg/tablet × 1000 bottles = 78,000,000 mg = 78,000 grams = 78 kg

   120 tablets/bottle × 500 mg/tablet × 1000 bottles = 60,000,000 mg = 60,000 grams = 60 kg

15. The density of mineral oil at 15°C is 0.76 g/mL and the density of water at the same temperature is 0.99 g/mL. What is the specific gravity of mineral oil?

$$\frac{0.76 \ g/mL}{0.99 \ g/mL} = 0.77$$

17. You measure out 32 grams of anhydrous ferrous sulfate, which has a density of 2.8 g/cm³. What volume will this amount of ferrous sulfate fill?

$32 \ g \div 2.8 \ g/cm^3 = 11.4 \ cm^3$

19. Jocelyn uses a graduated cylinder to measure 45 mL of an oral solution. The pharmacist tells her to draw the solution up in a 60-mL syringe instead, because it will be more accurate. When she draws the solution up into the syringe, she sees that the volume is 42 mL.

   a. What could account for the shortage?

   The accuracy of the syringe or the accuracy of the graduated cylinder could account for the shortage. A graduated cylinder is generally considered less accurate than a syringe.

   b. Assuming that all the solution made it into the syringe, what is the percent error of the graduated cylinder Jocelyn originally used?

   3 mL/42 mL = x/100 = 7.1%

21. At room temperature, 99% ethanol has a density of 0.83 g/mL. You have an 8-fluid ounce and a pint bottle. Which bottle will you choose to hold 265 g of ethanol?

   265 g ÷ 0.83 g/mL = 220 mL
   8 fl oz × 30 mL/fl oz = 240 mL; 1 pint = 16 fl oz or 480 mL. Therefore, use the 8-fl oz bottle.

23. The dermatologist orders the following ointment frequently for her patients with seborrheic dermatitis:

Precipitated sulfur	10 g
salicylic acid	2.5 g
water soluble ointment base	qs to 100 g

   a. How much of each ingredient is needed to make 1 kg of ointment?

   2.5 g/100 g = x/1 kg × 1 kg/1000 g x = 25 g salicylic acid
   10 g/100 g = y/1 kg × 1 kg/1000 g y = 100 g precipitated sulfur

   b. How much of each ingredient is necessary to make 454 grams?

   2.5 g/100 g = x/454 g x = 11.35 g salicylic acid
   10 g/100 g = y/454 g y = 45.4 g precipitated sulfur

25. The density of corn oil at room temperature is 0.92 g/mL. Of a quart, pint, and half-gallon capacity bottle, which would best contain the volume of 1 kg of corn oil?

   0.92 g/mL = 1000 g/x
   x = 1087 mL, requires ½ gal

Chapter 13

1. A vial of cefazolin for IV use is reconstituted with 45 mL of fluid and contains 50 mL of cefazolin 1 g/5 mL when correctly reconstituted.
   a. What volume does the dry powder displace?
      50 mL – 45 mL = 5 mL displaced by powder
   b. How many grams of cefazolin are in the vial?
      1 g/5 mL × 50 mL = 50 g/5 = 10 g
   c. To prepare a 2 g dose, what volume will be withdrawn?
      1 g/5 mL = 2 g/x
      x = 10 mL

3. The pharmacist prepares amoxicillin oral suspension that contains 500 mg/5 mL when correctly reconstituted. A full bottle contains 150 mL. How much amoxicillin is in a full bottle?
   500 mg/5 mL = x/150
   x = 15,000 mg or 15 g

5. Nurse Nancy calls you from the surgery unit to say that she mistakenly read the ceftriaxone reconstitution directions and added 5.6 mL lidocaine 1% instead of 3.6 mL. She is a new graduate and asks you what she should do. The ceftriaxone is for an IM injection in a woman who weighs 50 kg. You answer (choose the best answer):
   a. "I'm not certain. Let me look into it and call you back"
   b. "Let me get the pharmacist for you. Will you please hold?"
   c. "This medication is inexpensive, and it would be uncomfortable to inject 6 mL of fluid. I suggest you throw it away and start over."

   Although all three answers are correct, it is not within the pharmacy technician's scope of practice to provide answer C. If the nurse is in the middle of trying to prepare a medication, answer B, which should provide a faster response, is the best answer.

7. You receive a drug order for 5% dextrose in water 1000 mL, plus 30 mEq KCl. A vial of KCl contains 2 mEq KCl/ mL. What volume of KCl will you add to the 1000-mL bag?
   1 mL/2 mEq × 30 mEq = 15 mL

9. Normal saline contains 0.9% NaCl. How many mEq of sodium are there in a 100-mL bag of normal saline? Refer to Table 13-1 for equivalent weight of sodium chloride.
   15.4 mEq/100 mL NS

11. A patient receives one 50-mEq prefilled syringe of sodium bicarbonate IV during a code blue. One mEq of sodium bicarbonate weighs 84 mg. How many grams of sodium bicarbonate did the patient receive?
    1 mEq/84 mg = 50 mEq/x; x = 4200 mg or 4.2 g

13. Prefilled sodium bicarbonate syringes, made especially to use in cardiac and respiratory emergencies for infants and young children, contain 10 mL of 4.2% sodium bicarbonate.
    a. How many mEq of sodium bicarbonate are in a syringe?

    4.2% = 420 mg/10 mL × 1 mEq/84mg × 10 mL/syringe = 5 mEq/syringe

    b. How many mEq of sodium bicarbonate are in 1 mL of the solution?

    5 mEq/10 mL = 0.5 mEq/1 mL

15. A physician orders that a patient receive 3000 mL of TPN fluids in a day.
    a. How many mL/hr will the patient receive?

    3000 mL/24 hr = x/1 hr

    x = 125 mL, or 125 mL/hr rate

    b. The orders for the TPN are received and processed at 1700 hours. The next batch of IV solutions will be made in the morning and delivered at 0900 hours. How many bags will the technician need to make to last until morning?

    17 – 09 = 8 hours

    125 mL/hr × 8 hours = 1000 mL, or one L bag

17. The physician orders a 500-mL bag of fluid to run in over 4 hours. How many mL/minute will the patient receive?

    500 mL/4 hours = 125 mL/hr

    125 mL/hr × 1 hr/60 min = 2.1 mL/min

19. The ICU pharmacist calls the central pharmacy to get a dopamine drip made for a patient. The standard concentration for dopamine drips in your hospital is 1600 mcg/ mL. Dopamine is available as 40 mg/mL in a 5-mL vial. How much dopamine will you add to a 250-mL bag to achieve the standard concentration?

    1600 mcg/mL = 1.6 mg/ mL × 250 mL = 400 mg dopamine/250 mL bag

    40 mg/ mL = 400 mg/x

    x = 10 mL or 2 vials

21. A stat IV order is written for a dehydrated patient. The order reads "1000 mL NS + 20 KCl, run in over 4 hours, then 150 mL/hr for 6 hours, then 125 mL/hr." After 6 hours the above orders are discontinued. How much normal saline has the patient received after 6 hours?

    First 4 hours, 1000 mL, then 150 mL/hr × 2 hours = 1300 mL

23. The home health pharmacy prepares peripheral nutrition bags for 83-year-old Leanne Abed, who is recovering from burns she sustained when her kitchen caught fire. The IV infuses at a rate of 100 mL/hr. Mrs. Abed also receives antibiotics at midnight, 0600, 1200, and 1800. The TPN is turned off for 30 minutes every 6 hours while the antibiotics infuse. How much TPN does Mrs. Abed receive in 1 day?

    100 mL/hr × 24 hr/day = 2400 mL. However, the IV is turned off for 2 hours each day, so 2400 mL – 200 mL = 2200 mL/day

25. Insulin drips are used to treat a serious condition in patients with poorly controlled diabetes, called diabetic ketoacidosis. In your hospital, the standard concentration of an insulin drip is 1 unit/ mL in 100-mL bags. Patient Annie Sweet is in the ICU and an insulin drip is ordered. Annie

receives 8 units/hr for 4 hours, then 6 units/hr for 3 hours, and for the last 7 hours has received 5 units/hour. How much fluid is left in Annie's IV bag?

1 unit/ mL, so 8 units/hr = 8 mL/hr; 8 × 4hr = 32 mL; 6 mL/hr × 3hr = 18 mL; 5 mL/hr × 7 hr = 35 mL

Total used = 85 mL, 15 mL remaining.

Chapter 14

1. Joe's Pharmacy buys 30 Lipitor® 80-mg tablets for $175.00 and sells those 30 tablets for $190.00. What is Joe's gross profit on this transaction?
   $190.00 – $175.00 = $15.00

3. Good Neighbor Pharmacy buys 90 Naprosyn® 250-mg tablets for $16.00. Good Neighbor's markup rate on this item is 25%. What is Good Neighbor's selling price for 90 Naprosyn® 250-mg tablets?
   $16.00 + 0.25($16.00) = $20.00

5. Wholesale Rx Inc offers Best Pharmacy a 26% discount on Effexor® 25-mg tablets. The regular wholesale price for 120 Effexor® 25-mg tablets is $270.00. What price does Best Pharmacy pay for 120 Effexor® 25-mg tablets?
   $270.00 – 0.26($270.00) = $199.80

7. The regular price of Lipitor® 40 mg is $98.50 for 60 tablets. Joe gets a 14% discount when buying from the wholesaler Meds R Us.
   a. What price does Joe pay for 60 tablets of Lipitor® 40 mg?
      $98.50 – 0.14($98.50) = $84.71
   b. It costs Joe $3.00 to dispense 60 tablets. Joe sells the 60 tablets for $95.48. What is Joe's net profit on this sale?
      $95.48 – $84.71 – $3.00 = $7.77

9. The AWP for Actonel® 35 mg is $130.00 for 12 tablets. Joe's Pharmacy can purchase Actonel® 35 mg for $115.00 for 12 tablets. It costs the pharmacy $2.00 to dispense the tablets.
   a. How much does it cost Joe's Pharmacy to fill a prescription for 12 Actonel® 35-mg tablets?
      $115.00 + $2.00 = $117.00
   b. The customer's insurance company will reimburse the pharmacy AWP + 3% + $2.00 dispensing fee. How much does the insurance company pay the pharmacy?
      $130.00 + 0.03($130.00) + $2.00 = $135.90
   c. What is the pharmacy's profit in this transaction?
      $135.90 – $117.00 = $18.90

11. The AWP for Levoxyl® 100 mcg is $54.00 for 100 tablets.
    a. What is the AWP per tablet?

    $$\frac{\$54.00}{100} = \$0.54$$

    b. What is the AWP for 30 Levoxyl® 100-mcg tablets?

    $$\frac{\$0.54}{tablet} \times 30 \ tablets = \$16.20$$

13. In January, the staff at Joe's Pharmacy performs an inventory and discovers that the value of the inventory is $75,000.00. Six months later another inventory is performed and the value is $60,000.00. What is the average inventory?

$$\frac{\$75,000 + \$60,000}{2} = \$67,500 \text{ average inventory}$$

15. In January, the staff at Joe's Pharmacy performs an inventory and discovers that the value of the inventory is $80,000.00. Six months later another inventory is performed and the value is $100,000.00. Over the course of a year, Joe spends $360,000.00 purchasing items to sell at the pharmacy.
    a. Find the average inventory value and the turnover rate.

    $90,000.00 = inventory value

    turnover rate = 4

    b. How long does it take to "turn over" the inventory?

    3 months

17. In January, the inventory value at Tom's Pharmacy is $125,000.00. Six months later the inventory value is $120,000.00. Over the course of a year, Tom spends $367,500.00 on items to sell. How long does it take to "turn over" the inventory at Tom's?

$$\frac{\$125,000 + \$120,000}{2} = \$122,500 \text{ average inventory}$$

Turnover rate = annual expenditures/average inventory

$$\frac{\$367,500}{\$122,500} = 3 \text{ turns per year, or every 4 months}$$

19. Neighborhood Pharmacy buys new compounding software for $350.00. The estimated lifetime of the software is 5 years. The disposal value of the software is $0. Find the annual depreciation for the software.

    Annual depreciation = total investment (cost) – disposal value/estima

$$\frac{\$350 - \$0}{5 \text{ years}} = \$70.00/\text{year depreciation}$$

21. Neighborhood Pharmacy invests in a new computer system at a cost of $12,000 for hardware and software. The life expectancy of their purchase is 6 years. The disposal value is estimated to be $750.00. Find the annual depreciation for their purchase.

$$\frac{\$12,000 - \$750}{6 \text{ years}} = \$1,875/\text{year}$$

23. The regular wholesale price for Enditch Ointment is $5.25/ounce. Ralph buys Enditch Ointment from Prescriptions R Us for $4.00/ounce.
    a. What is the discount offered by Prescriptions R Us?

    $5.25 – $4.00 = $1.25

b. What is the discount rate offered by Prescriptions R Us?

$$\frac{\$1.25}{\$5.25} \times 100\% = 24\%$$

25. **Blue Shield reimburses Small's Pharmacy AWP plus a $7.50 professional fee for filling a generic prescription. The AWP for 100 furosemide 40-mg tablets is $17.80. Bud buys 100 furosemide tablets for $14.90, and his costs for filling the prescription is $3.25.**

a. What is Bud's profit when a patient has Blue Shield Insurance?

Bud's costs = $14.90 + $3.25 = $18.15

Blue Shield pays $17.80 + $7.50 = $25.30

Bud's profits = reimbursement − cost = $25.30 − $18.15 = $7.15

b. Bud usually sells 100 furosemide tablets for $24.50. How much less is Bud's profit than in part a?

Bud's costs = $18.15

Bud's receipts on 100 furosemide 40 mg = $24.50

Bud's usual profit = $24.50 − $18.15 = $6.35

Bud's profit is $0.80 less.

Index